...to thank the people wh...

Chance, Necessity, Love

Chance, Necessity, Love

An Evolutionary Theology of Cancer

Leonard M. Hummel

Gayle E. Woloschak

FOREWORD BY
Deanna Thompson

CASCADE *Books* · Eugene, Oregon

CHANCE, NECESSITY, LOVE
An Evolutionary Theology of Cancer

Cascade Books
An Imprint of Wipf and Stock Publishers
199 W. 8th Ave., Suite 3
Eugene, OR 97401

www.wipfandstock.com

PAPERBACK ISBN: 978-1-4982-8453-0
HARDCOVER ISBN: 978-1-4982-8455-4
EBOOK ISBN: 978-1-4982-8454-7

Cataloguing-in-Publication data:

Names: Hummel, Leonard M. | Woloschak, Gayle E.

Title: Chance, necessity, love : an evolutionary theology of cancer / Leonard M.
Hummel and Gayle E. Woloschak.

Description: Eugene, OR: Cascade Books, 2017 | Includes bibliographical refer-
ences and index.

Identifiers: ISBN 978-1-4982-8453-0 (paperback) | ISBN 978-1-4982-8455-4 (hard-
cover) | ISBN 978-1-4982-8454-7 (ebook)

Subjects: LCSH: 1. Cancer. | 2. Cancer History. | 3. Practical Theology. | I. Title.

Classification: RC275 C35 2017 (print) | RC275 (ebook)

Manufactured in the U.S.A.   07/17/17

Figure 1 reproduced by permission from Mel Greaves, *Cancer: The Evolutionary
Legacy* (Oxford: Oxford University Press, 2001), Figure 23.1, 214.

Contents

Foreword

When it comes to cancer, we often use military metaphors to describe our relationship to the disease. Those with cancer are called on to fight it bravely; those who die from cancer have "lost their battle" with the disease. We wear ribbons, sign up for relays, and pledge our support in the fight against cancer.

But Augustus, one of the main characters in *The Fault in Our Stars*, John Green's popular novel about teenagers living with cancer, makes clear why the military images often fall short. "What am I at war with?" he asks. "My cancer. And what is my cancer? My cancer is me. The tumors are made of me. They're made of me as surely as my brain and my heart are made of me."[1]

In their theology of cancer, theologian Leonard Hummel and scientist Gayle Woloschak are after "faithful understandings" of cancer in order to envision "wise responses" to this quintessential disease of life. They begin with the science of Augustus's claim: how cancer arises from the very fiber of our being, and how those very same evolutionary forces of chance and necessity that make it possible for creatures to continue to adapt and survive also allow cancer to emerge within the fibers of our being.

But if cancer—a disease that causes great harm and suffering—is constitutive of our being, we are left with a host of theological questions about a God who creates and sustains a creation that opens up to the chance and

---

1. John Green, *The Fault in Our Stars*, New York: Penguin, Reprint Edition, 2014, 216.

necessity of cancer. The heart of Hummel and Woloschak's project is to contemplate those questions and offer wise responses that can help us come to terms with the realities of cancer alongside affirmations that the God who creates and sustains is One who loves and cares for creation.

One of the strengths of this project is the authors' careful consideration of not just one but multiple possible wise theological responses to the evolutionary inevitability of cancer. Hummel and Woloschak consider theologies of acceptance that posit a good God as creator of evolutionary processes where chaos, suffering, and tragedy cannot be avoided. They also explore theologies of hope determined to hold on to a vision of God who lovingly redeems and heals a world full of such suffering.

Their refusal to side only with acceptance or just with hope is the most compelling aspect of Hummel and Woloschak's work. As someone who lives with incurable cancer, I find the space in between acceptance and hope to be more realistic and helpful than the battlefield where I must wage war. That cancer is "made of me" suggests an acceptance of sorts—of trying to figure out what it means to live *with* this part of my being. At the same time, that cancer brings so much pain and suffering into my life and the lives of so many others engenders a longing, a hope that God will bring about a future of less suffering, less harm.

Even as Woloschak and Hummel understand cancer as an evolutionary inevitability of chance and necessity, they point to ways in which scientific advances are "taming chance" through the development of new treatments, signs of hope that the force of cancer can be diminished. But ours remains a world where cancer lives, a world in need of more meditations like Hummel and Woloschak's about how our theologies might help us make meaning of life with cancer and of a God present in the midst of it.

Deanna A. Thompson

Holy Week 2017
Saint Paul, Minnesota

Preface

What exactly is cancer? And where is God and what is love amidst the disease of cancer? The purpose of this book is to address these questions. In order to do so, we first clarify a number of scientific complexities about cancer. Next, we consider a variety of compelling theological perspectives regarding the nature of this disease. In light of these perspectives, we conclude with proposals for what both cannot and can be changed about cancers. We reveal cancer to be an evolutionary disease that develops according to the same dynamics of chance (that is, random occurrences) and necessity (law-like regularities) at work in all evolutionary phenomena.

Therefore, we ask throughout these questions: where is God and what is love within the evolutionary chance and necessity operative in all dimensions of cancer? We offer the following responses: (1) the evolving work of scientific communities to understand and to find better ways to respond to the disease of cancer is itself the work of God amidst this evolutionary phenomenon; (2) through our efforts to make theological sense of the chance and necessity that drive the evolution of cancers, we may discern divine love in, with, and under these evolutionary dynamics. In making the above claims, we also propose that comprehending how cancer is a product of biological evolution and then grappling with God's place in that process will assist us in developing faithful understandings about and wise responses to cancers.

How does the book accomplish this?

First, it makes the disease of cancer comprehensible—that is, a phenomenon whose essential features we may grasp. It does so by highlighting the red thread of evolutionary chance and necessity that runs throughout the onset and development of all cancers. To be sure, this book does not attempt to describe this disease exhaustively, and therefore should not be used as a manual for cancer diagnosis or cancer care. But it does lay out the key components of cancer, even as it highlights the complexities at work in all of its occurrences.

Second, the book grapples theologically with the place of God and the role of love in a disease that evolves through the interplay of random occurrences and lawlike regularities. In doing so, it addresses these questions: how may God be said to be "good" if the development of life and the development of cancer are linked by common evolutionary processes? What abilities and responsibilities do we have in the face of cancer?

Third, the book proposes that our seeking both scientific and faithful understandings about the disease of cancer may reveal and make real the love of God amidst its evolutionary chance and necessity. In the concluding chapters, we offer examples of how divine love shows itself in those theologies that communicate God's care for this world and in scientific research that enables us to better cope with the chance and necessity of cancer.

Our focus is on the basic science of the disease of cancer and how to come to religious terms with its very existence. That is, unlike many other works about religion and cancer, we do not center our inquiry on the experience of illness by persons with cancer, but rather on the experience of all humanity given the persistence of this disease. Therefore, our book is not meant to replace or compete with the many outstanding in print and online resources now available to guide persons with cancer and their families who are facing diagnosis and treatment.

Nor does this book offer a series of "cancer facts" about any particular kind of cancer. Nor is its description of cancers intended to be directly applicable to any particular case of cancer. Rather, through this book we intend to provide our primary audience—religious leaders and all persons with inquiring minds—with a general knowledge of the disease and some theological perspectives on it. In doing so, we have attempted to provide the most accurate and up-to-date findings about cancer. But we also caution our readers to remember, as our review of the history of cancer research indicates, that findings that were once thought to be accurate and robust have sometimes proven not to be, and that what is "up-to-date" about cancer changes almost daily. Expressing this caution, we also express the hope that this work will enable readers to grasp what is essential in current concepts about cancer, and thereby assist them to comprehend new findings as they become available.

The authors, Gayle Woloschak and Leonard Hummel, met in summer 2007 at the annual assembly of the Association of Teaching Theologians of the Evangelical Lutheran Church in America. There, Leonard shared his interest in ideas about chance, necessity, and love in the thought of Charles Sanders Peirce as they might bear on the study of cancer. In response, Gayle mentioned that she had a forthcoming article in *Zygon* entitled "Chance and Necessity in Arthur Peacocke's Scientific Work," which demonstrated the connection between Peacocke's work on cancer and his religious thinking!

The authors represent diverse disciplines of study. Gayle is a wet-bench scientist with a working lab that revolves around cancer research in a variety of different projects, including developing tools and approaches to better diagnose and treat cancer. She has been involved in the science-religion dialogue for well over two decades, predominantly because of the need for understanding and openness on all sides of the discussion. Leonard comes to this work as a practical theologian concerned with bringing religious understandings to questions and problems of human being, so that humans might respond with faithful understandings and wise practices.

Even with our different professional orientations, it was obvious to both of us in coming together and planning for this book that we share many convictions and hopes. We believe that scientific knowledge—while it is always a construct of cultures, and therefore always subject to cultural criticisms, and that it too often is misused by those with power—is a God-given means to help humankind to understand the nature of creation. In particular, we believe that attending to evolutionary theory is not just a way to honor scientists and their endeavors, but it also is a means by which we may reveal and make real God's good purposes for creation. We hold that evolutionary theory affords us insights into the nature of cancer and care for those suffering with it—and thereby is a tool with which we may do the work of the Lord.

Acknowledgments

All scholarly endeavors emerge from communities of inquiry, without which their fruits would not be possible. I, Leonard, would like to acknowledge the generous support of the Lutheran Theological Seminary at

Gettysburg, in particular the oversight of President Michael Cooper-White and Dean Robin Steinke. They encouraged me to teach three distinct courses on cancer and religion during my years there, and granted me sabbatical to work on this book. In the conception and execution of this project, I have enjoyed the enduring encouragement and insight of Dr. Eric H. Crump. Eric has brought his systematic and historical theological acumen to bear on its complexities, especially on the philosophical origins and religious implications of the concepts of chance, necessity, and love.

I am very grateful to Ann Pederson, Professor of Religion, Augustana College, Sioux Falls, South Dakota, whose own interest in science and religion studies as they bear on cancer stimulated my thinking. Her careful and helpful reading of texts—especially as they relate to Peacocke's thought on chance, necessity, and religion—has been a boon to this project. Furthermore, Ann's arranging for me to present portions of this text to faculty and students at Augustana in January of 2012, in January of 2013, and again in January of 2014 provided important feedback for this work while it was in progress.

From his endeavors as a systematic theologian who has focused on evolutionary phenomena of various sorts and on the larger question of how to integrate science and theology in theological education, Ronald Cole-Turner of Pittsburg Theological Seminary has served as a helpful guide. He has pointed out the significance of our work on cancer and religion for seminary education. I am indebted to Chris Schlauch of Boston University for his careful read of this text and subsequent empathy for all of us struggling to make sense of sources of suffering and sources of compassion in a world with cancer in it. I am also grateful for the enduring and heartfelt interest of Deanna Thompson of Hamline University.

I would like to thank the Louisville Institute for awarding me a Grant for Researchers in 2012–2013, for my project "The Very Fiber of Our Being: A Pastoral Theology of Cancer and Evolution." That enabled me to work with pastors to explore the significance of cancer as a phenomenon of evolution for their congregational ministry.

Finally, I would like to express my gratitude for the contributions by the late Edward Farley for his conversations with me about my plans for a practical theology of cancer during the period when I was on faculty of Vanderbilt Divinity School and Ed was the Drucilla Moore Buffington Professor of Theology, Emeritus, at Vanderbilt. Ed gave much time and attention to my work—and, on my behalf, composed a short, unpublished piece "Some Preliminary Thoughts on a Practical Theology of Cancer," that we cite in this book.

I, Gayle, would foremost like to thank the members of the Orthodox Church community that have helped to shape my thinking and taught me the value of tension and disagreement in understanding issues. These include the members of the Social and Moral Issues Commission of SCOBA, the LOGOS group, the members and conferences of the Orthodox Theological Society of America, the members and conferences of the Orthodox Christian Association of Medicine Psychology and Religion, and the Sophia Institute. I would like to thank the people who contributed to the inquiries and discussions that informed this work, several of whom are also in Leonard's list of acknowledgements, especially Eric Crump, Ronald Cole-Turner, and Ann Pederson.

I am grateful for the input of Dr. Tatjana Paunesku at Northwestern University, my colleague and long-time collaborator; my many colleagues at the Zygon Center and Lutheran School of Theology at Chicago who over the years have shared provocative perspectives and insights; my students at Lutheran School of Theology at Chicago, Pittsburgh Theological Seminary, and St. Vladimir's Orthodox Seminary who have made me think and rethink my ideas. Finally, I wish to thank my bishops His Beatitude Metropolitan Constantine of blessed memory, His Eminence Archbishop Antony, and His Grace Bishop Daniel of the Ukrainian Orthodox Church of the USA. Their trust and faith have guided and inspired me to continue on my quest for a better understanding of the science-religion interface. Finally, both Leonard and I are grateful to the Association of Theological Schools for awarding us a Collaborative Scholars Grant for "Chance, Necessity, Love: An Evolutionary Theology of Cancer" (2012–2013).

Both Gayle and Leonard express deep and special thanks to Aaron Smith, PhD, for his careful proofreading and editing of our text for submission to Cascade Press. Aaron holds a PhD in systematic theology and was assistant professor of theology before becoming a candidate for rostered ministry in the ELCA.

Introduction

Background of *Chance, Necessity, Love:*
An Evolutionary Theology of Cancer

C ancer is a disease replete with paradox. On the one hand, it touches the
lives of both the more powerful and the less powerful. On the other
hand, differences in cancer vulnerability do occur through occasionally inherited predispositions to the disease and through the ways that economic
and social inequalities generally affect its incidence and outcome. Cancer
also is a disease that may or may not be treated successfully depending on
the stage of its detection and on the treatment and aggressiveness of the
disease. Furthermore, many kinds of cancers have always been with us and
may always be with us. Still, the occurrence of certain cancers may be affected by individual and social efforts, and new treatments for care and cure
have been and continue to be developed. Therefore, the following assertion
is puzzling but it is also quite true: cancer is something that both cannot
and can be changed.

The underlying reason for this paradox may be located in the nature of
the disease itself: cancer progresses—or more accurately, evolves—through
the complex interplay of chance occurrences and the lawlike regularities
that govern the outcome of those occurrences. That is, just as DNA mutations and natural selection for those mutations are involved in the evolution
of various species, so also mutational mechanisms and forces of selection
are at work in the evolution of individual cancers. This may be said another way and with a more ironic emphasis: while operations of chance and

1

necessity promote the evolution of life, so those very same forces drive the evolution of a disease that may end lives.

Cancer is a disease whose origin and progression often vex and confuse cancer patients and those who care for them. Those diagnosed with the disease often struggle to understand its possible causes and future course. Family members wonder what they must accept and may hope for. Pastors hear much about cancer: newly suspected causes, new possible cures, and new dangers in treatment—and then pray and hope for their people. The evolutionary chance and necessity at work in the onset and development of cancer may perplex all people about what can be changed and what cannot be changed about this disease.

Much of the confusion in comprehending these aspects of cancer arises from the complex origins and development of the disease. Consider the figure below, which diagrams both the lawlike regularities involved in the evolution of cancer, as well as representing, in the gaming metaphors of a roulette wheel and "full house," the role of chance in that evolution.

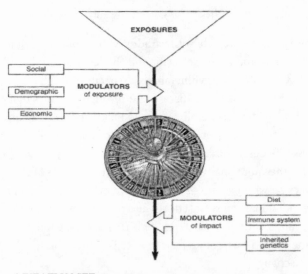

MUTATION SET

Inherited → IIIIIIIIIIIIIIIIIIIIIIIIIIIIIIIIIIIIIIIIIIIIIIIII → FULL HOUSE
CLONAL ESCAPE

Mutation   TIME

Figure 1: A prescription for composite risk of cancer (reproduced with permission from Mel Greaves, *Cancer: The Evolutionary Legacy*. Oxford: Oxford University Press, 2001, Figure 23.1, 214).

Later in our work, we will review this graphic. However, even a cursory look at the "cancer facts" in this figure may lead people of faith to ask this question: how does God figure in—that is, where is God in the world of cancer that is shaped by the chance and necessity portrayed in it?

In this book, we will address these questions of life and death—of living with a world with cancer in it—and, in doing so, make recommendations for faithful understandings and wise practices. In making these recommendations, this book will situate itself within the field of practical theology.

Practical Theology as Interpreting Situations for Faithful Understandings and Wise Response

The constructive theologian Edward Farley offered a simple definition of practical theology as "a theological interpretation of a situation."[1] While Farley's definition is not strictly endorsed by all practical theologians, it does describe how many of them carry out their inquiry. Works in practical theology have focused on a variety of situations including women and poverty, the coping strategies of Lutherans in the United States, the struggles of ordained Southern Baptist women, a theology of and for disabled persons, and many others.[2] A common feature of practical theological endeavors is their bringing theological insights to bear on these and other circumstances so that persons of faith and religious communities may respond with faithful understandings—those that contribute to right relationship with God—and wise responses—those that contribute to human flourishing.

The very occurrence of cancer has long been a "situation" of humanity, a phenomenon that persons with the disease, persons caring for those with the disease, and all of humanity have confronted. Furthermore, the history of the disease reflects the complexity encountered throughout time and across cultures of attempts to detect the disease and to make meaning of its occurrences.[3] Still, some summaries may be made of those complexi-

1. Farley, "Interpreting Situations," 118–27.

2. For example, see Campbell-Reed, "Baptist Clergywomen's Narratives," Schaller, "Resisting Stares and Stereotypes," Hummel, *Clothed in Nothingness*, and Couture, *Blessed Are the Poor?*

3. Furthermore, the disease of cancer constitutes a piece of natural history. Mostly absent among invertebrates, its spread throughout vertebrate life is uneven. For example, its incidence is much higher among domesticated mammals than those of the same species in the wild (Capasso, "Antiquity of Cancer"; Weiss, "Early Concepts of Cancer").

ties. For example, it is not clear whether the early Mesopotamians and the ancient Egyptians conceived of it as a distinct disease process.[4] On the other hand, cases of esophageal cancer in China have been recorded for thousands of years. And it is quite clear that an extensive array of cancers were recognized in Indian Ayurvedic medical writings.

Much of the current cancer basic science that crosses contemporary cultures has developed from refinements of and in reaction to speculations about this disorder in ancient Greece and Rome. Believing that the human body was composed of constantly shifting proportions of four humors (phlegm, blood, yellow bile, and black bile), Hippocrates (460–377 BCE) had concluded that cancer resulted from an overexpression of black bile. His theory arose in response to the alleged dark hue of some breast tumors—the most diagnosed cancers throughout antiquity and the early modern period.[5] The name Hippocrates devised to describe the disease, "karkinos" or "crab"—because tumors seemed to him to have branching legs like that animal—has stuck both as a designation for all occurrences of cancer and for its predominant manifestation in the epithelial linings of organs (i.e., "carcinomas").

The title of one work on this history, *From Demons and Evil Spirits to Cancer Genes: The Development of Concepts Concerning the Causes of Cancer and Carcinogenesis*, reveals how religious metaphors have arisen in response to our attempts to understand the origins of cancer.[6] And the very title of a recent major best seller, *The Emperor of All Maladies: A Biography of Cancer*, suggests that this life-threatening disease has something like a life of its own, and may, with profit, be reflected upon as a thing unto itself.[7] In this clearly and wonderfully written telling of the near history of human understandings of and treatments for cancer, Siddhartha Mukherjee notes how reflecting on the inner life of cancer led him to regard it as having something like a personality of its own: "I started imagining my project as a 'history' of cancer. But it felt, inescapably, as if I were writing not about

---

Archaeology offers little solid evidence, since the soft tissues in which most cancers occur are usually not well preserved (Fitzgerald, *From Demons and Evil Spirits*, 5–7). Nevertheless, findings of sarcomas—cancers that arise in connective tissues and bones— among dinosaurs and ancient homo-sapiens testify to its antiquity (Capasso, "Antiquity of Cancer").

4. Fitzgerald, *From Demons and Evil Spirits*; Weiss, "Early Concepts of Cancer."

5. Rather, *The Genesis of Cancer.*

6. Fitzgerald, *From Demons and Evil Spirits.*

7. Mukherjee, *The Emperor of All Maladies.*

some*thing* but about some*one*."[8] Accordingly, Mukherjee does not shy away from offering colorful and evocative descriptions the disease:

> This image—of cancer as our desperate, malevolent, contemporary doppelgaenger—is so haunting because it is at least partly true. Susan Sontag warned against overburdening an illness with metaphors. But this is not a metaphor. Down to their innate molecular core, cancer cells are hyperactive, survival-endowed, scrappy, fecund, inventive copies of ourselves.[9]

These metaphorically rich descriptions of cancer arise out of scientifically precise accounts of its evolutionary processes. "If we, as a species, are the ultimate product of Darwinian selection, then so, too, is this incredible disease that lurks inside us."[10]

Some scientific analyses of cancer have crossed the border of metaphorical descriptions of its operations into straightforward religious language about its nature. In 1928, William H. Woglom, a leading researcher with Britain's Imperial Cancer Research Fund, wrote an article in *The Atlantic Monthly* that bore this striking title: "Cancer, the Scourge of God."[11] Woglom began his essay with this provocative description: "The cancer cell, to borrow a phrase from Schopenhauer, has the will to live. That is to say, it is able to defy those forces which restrain the multiplication of normal cells and so preserve a just proportion among the various parts of the organism"[12] Nowhere in this article's review of cancer knowledge in that era are religious matters discussed. Yet, given the title of Woglum's article and its leading sentence, certainly some readers may be left wondering what religious sense may be brought to the situation of cancer—e. g., what might be the will of God in relationship to the will of cancer cells?

Again: the purpose of this book is to bring theological understandings to the situation of cancer for both faithful understandings and wise practices. We next shall explicate what we intend through such goals.

By faithful understandings, we mean those that reflect on and promote trust in God and in God's purposes in a world with cancer in it. Here is another way to say this: in this theology of cancer, we shall reflect on God's ways for the world. Such faithful inquiry into a world with cancer

8. Ibid., 39.
9. Ibid., 38, 388.
10. Ibid., 39.
11. Woglum, "Cancer," 806–12.
12. Ibid., 806.

in it does leave much room for wonder, and this openness is evidenced in the questions we posed in the preface (i.e., where is God and what is love within the evolutionary chance and necessity at work in all dimensions of cancer?), and also from those that we will ask throughout the book. Therefore we do not seek to provide conclusive answers in this book to many of the questions we pose, but we do engage a "community of inquiry"—the thoughts and ideas of other believers—in order to address these questions.

The speculations of the nineteenth-century American philosopher, Charles Sanders Peirce, provide the source for the following summary of our approach to questions like the ones we are bringing to this practical theology of the disease of cancer.

While we never obtain certain understanding of ourselves, the world, or God, Peirce maintains that we may participate in a community of inquirers who can help us achieve a better understanding of all of them. Knowing that, and knowing that there are only provisional answers to life's larger questions—or, in some cases, no apparent answers, but only the process of our careful asking—perhaps that is, for now, the answer to them.

By wise responses, we mean those that, in their engagement with the structures of the world, enable one to live in it both productively and well. We find inspiration for this notion of wisdom within the broader purpose of biblical wisdom literature. In a recent work, Hebrew Bible scholar James Crenshaw defines this wisdom as "the attempt to cope with reality as it presents itself in real life."[13] He also proposes that the most encompassing feature of wisdom's legacy "is its *ability to cope* with reality, be it favorable or threatening."[14]

As indicated by engaging Peirce, we find these perspectives on wisdom in Hebrew Scriptures to be commensurable with the goal of practical inquiry in classical American pragmatism. One description of Peirce's thought, offered by John E. Smith, provides a good summary of the practical bearings of intellectual inquiries like ours:

> The whole . . . apparatus of man [sic] comes into play in order to cope. . . . This is what Peirce and the pragmatists meant when they said that thought is practical; it is a means of extricating us from

13. Crenshaw, *Old Testament Wisdom*, 7. It is interesting to note that in Gerhard Von Rad's classic work on wisdom literature, the chapter describing the various proverbs which assume an orderly universe is translated into English as "The Essentials for Coping with Reality." See von Rad, *Wisdom in Israel*.

14. Ibid., 230. Emphasis added.

our predicaments and, at the same time, of reshaping as much of the environment as is within our power in order to destroy the factors in the universe that work against our well-being and even our very survival.[15]

For theological reasons that we shall later elaborate, we endorse scientific understandings of cancer as instruments given us by God with which we may both comprehend the environment out of which the disease emerges and, to a degree, also reshape it.[16] That is, we believe that these understandings make available to us, more or less, "reality as it presents itself in the real world" and, thereby, with tools to help us cope with it.[17]

Accordingly, in this theology of cancer, we shall detail scientific findings about cancer and then bring theological perspectives to bear on them in order to recommend responses that may assist us in facing cancer as a force that may threaten our well-being and survival. In doing so, we will draw on insights from the burgeoning literature in religion and science, especially that which deals with theology and evolution. However, as a practical theological endeavor, our inquiry will distinguish itself from most of these works by directing its questions concerning both theological understandings of evolution and of the particular evolutionary phenomena of cancer toward questions of their significance for faithful understandings and wise responses.

Our Path through This Book

Through this book, we will both introduce the reader to the complexities of basic cancer science in a clear and compelling manner and introduce various evolutionary theologies of the disease that will assist the reader to receive the science of the disease with acceptance, hope, and love.

The rationale for the structure of this book was suggested by the findings of two focus groups with clergy and laypersons, who graciously offered their best thoughts on what might be the contents for a course in a practical

---

15. Smith, *The Spirit of American Philosophy*, 21.

16. We own that scientific knowledge is a social construct. And we recognize that social forces both facilitate and hinder the acquisition and distribution of the findings of scientific inquiry.

17. Smith, *The Spirit of American Philosophy*, 7.

theology of cancer.[18] The members of both groups were unanimous in wanting to learn about the disease process of cancer:

> "Knowing the language of cancer—it's ever changing because of the research taking place. That might help the caregiver understand the level of hope that there is or the level of compassion that needs to be there because of the seriousness of it." "I want to know what it is; we want to have at least a basic understanding of what it is just so that that's a way of beginning to deal with it or help somebody else to deal with it, just to have a better idea of what it is."

The other area of consensus among these caregivers was the need for a theology about cancer itself:

> "Just the theology of life and death and what we all face and cancer . . . . This is the real stuff." "But often they [cancer patients] look for reasons: 'Is God trying to teach me something? Am I being punished? What is God trying to tell me through this?' So then we get into some theological questions as to the cause and the 'whys' of why things happen in life?" "A theology that it's an imperfect world . . . ." "Big theological questions about suffering and evil and how illness fits into those questions."

The participants then concurred that such a theology might make for better congregational care of cancer patients and for better congregational responses to the disease of cancer itself. Congruent with these two major findings, this book focuses on the basic science of cancer in its first section, and, in its second section, offers a practical theology of cancer.

We begin our first section with the chapter, "The Very Fiber of our Being: Cancer as a Disease of Cells." Here, we introduce current science about cancer cells and all cells that, although it is a basic science, also reveals a profound irony: while cancers destroy cells, the very fiber of our being, cancers themselves also are nothing other than the very fiber of our being—normal cells gone awry. Accordingly, we detail the ways in which cancers are diseases of cells, the constitutive elements of life that, in their development, may destroy these very elements.

In the chapter that follows, "Chance and Necessity in Life: Cancer as a Disease of Genes," we describe how cancer cells originate from and develop according to the same molecular activities of genes that may occur within all non-cancerous cells. In doing so, we reveal how the nature and

---

18. Hummel, "A Thing That Cannot and Can Be Changed."

operations of genes provide a simultaneously unifying and highly complex explanation for the causes and the very nature of cancers.

In the final chapter of this section, "Hallmarks of Oncological Development: Cancer as an Evolutionary Disease," we describe how this disease of cells and genes develops in real time according to Darwinian evolutionary dynamics of random variation and natural selection. As we do so, we focus on six hallmarks of this development that constitute the key features of its onset and that, considered together, reveal cancers to be hardy and robust "survivors" in a world of evolutionary chance and necessity. Having concluded that cancer is a disease of evolution, we also shall conclude this chapter and this first section by noting the consequent need for a practical theology of cancer for faithful understandings of and wise responses to the existence and persistence of this evolutionary phenomenon.

In the second section of this book, we begin to develop a practical theology with the chapter, "'No Exclusion of Chaos and Suffering:' Acceptance in a World with Cancers." Here, we consider one faithful theological understanding that proposes that God has created a world in which there must be cancers and that, consequently, recommends the wise response of our accepting this fact so that we might develop empathy for this world and for those who suffer from cancers. Accordingly, this chapter offers a perspective on evolution that calls on us to accept that, given evolutionary processes, various forms of natural suffering, including various kinds of cancers, are inevitable.

In the chapter that follows, "Something More: Hope in a World of Cancer Chance and Necessity," we examine another and different perspective on cancer that may be summarized this way: God has something better in mind, or has a promise of something more, than this world with cancers in them. While we will conclude that theological proposals attempting to describe a cancer-free time to come show themselves upon analysis to be incoherent, we also will review ways in which we may still hope in God's promise to deliver us from the sufferings of cancer.

Even with the differences among some of the theological positions described in these first two chapters, we note how both propose that cancers come about through the processes of evolutionary chance and necessity and how both understand that the love of God makes possible their recommended responses of acceptance and hope. Accordingly, in the chapter that follows, "Chance, Necessity, Love: A Theology of Cancer," we examine more closely the concepts of "chance" and "necessity" themselves in three major evolutionary thinkers, for the insights into how we might discern love—both divine and human—to be at work in a world with cancers. We conclude that the love of God may be understood to be operative in, with, and under the evolution of cancers in two ways: (1) through scientific endeavors that help us to comprehend and, sometimes, to cut into their evolutionary development; and (2) through symbols and stories that testify to the love of God amidst their evolutionary chance and necessity.

In the conclusion, we focus on the benefits for theological understanding and the care of souls that accrue from considering cancer to be a phenomenon of evolution. We review and make recommendations for continued studies in practical theology and pastoral theology that may witness to the love of God in a world with the evolutionary chance and necessity of cancers.

Final Introductory Remarks

Cancer is an outcome of biological evolution arising through mechanisms driven by chance and necessity. In light of various theologies that take evolutionary biology into account, how may love—divine and human—be discerned amidst these evolutionary mechanisms? One answer is this:

> Through their research, scientific "communities of inquiry" strive to understand and, increasingly, succeed at understanding the evolutionary nature of cancers. The efforts of these communities, carried out by persons both of faith and of no faith, may evidence the love of God at work in, with, and under the evolution of cancers.

Another answer is this:

> Through symbols and stories about the chance and necessity of the disease of cancer, we have the ability to construct meanings about that evolutionary phenomenon. God may work in, with, and under these constructions to reveal and make real God's love for this world with cancers in it.

The central argument of this book is this: that comprehending how cancer is a product of biological evolutionary processes, and then grappling with how we may understand God's love given these processes, will assist religious communities and individual believers to develop faithful understandings about and wise responses to cancer.

Cancer: An Evolutionary Disease of Chance and Necessity

Chapter 1

The Very Fiber of Our Being:
Cancer as a Disease of Cells

Introduction and Perspectives

In 2006, Walter Wangerin, a Lutheran pastor and theologian, was diagnosed with lung cancer. After he received this news and began treatment, Wangerin wrote a memoir of his diary and letters that he later published. In his book, Wangerin described his inner world, his relationships with others, and the events unfolding around his cancer with an irony, beauty, bite, and grace familiar to those accustomed to his many other works. Wangerin detailed much—his treatments, his doubts, struggles, disappointments, and his hopes—and placed all within the frame of his faith in the enduring goodness of God.

Most of Wangerin's reflections focus on his illness—that is, on the sorrows and joys concomitant with his coping with cancer. However, some of his meditations are on the disease itself, and on the relationship between his body and that disease as he lives in the "meantime" between his diagnosis and whatever the outcome of that may be. He writes: "I recognize this [his living in this meantime] in all the fibers of my being, for these are they who have communicated corruption to me. *All the fibers of my being*."[1]

---

1. Wangerin Jr., *Letters*, 160.

Wangerin seems to sense that his body and his disease are one or that they are of the same stock—himself. "Cancer is tissue which is in company with all my other tissues—*all my fibers!*"[2]

Cancer, Wangerin asserts, is of his own fiber, and in doing so he employs a metaphor that is also quite accurate. In plant biology, a fiber is a cell with thick walls separating it from other similar cells. By extension, the metaphorical meaning of fiber is of something's "essential character; basic strength or toughness; fortitude."[3] As we shall see in this chapter, Wangerin is quite right. Cancer *is* our fiber—for the very constitutive element of all life is the cell and cancer cells are nothing other than our own cells. Wangerin's use of the metaphor of "fiber" also seems reflective of his own fiber— his strength of character: "perhaps that phrase may touch upon my reasons for refusing to use the imagery of warfare when speaking of my cancer. I have never construed my cancer as my enemy."[4] However, there are other accounts of cancer, some of which emphasize not so much acceptance of the disease, but both recount and call for struggle with it—even if those accounts employ some of the very same terms that Wangerin does.

In 1726, Peregrine Laziosi (1260–1345) was canonized as Saint Peregrine. Born in Forli, Italy, Peregrine was, by all accounts, a bad Catholic in his early years who later repented and became a highly ascetic believer. Diagnosed with cancer of the foot, the following is one account of his reception of grace:

> A huge ulcerative growth appeared on Peregrine's leg . . . . [T]he best physicians . . . pronounced the lesion to be cancerous and advised amputation of the leg. The night before the scheduled operation, Peregrine dragged himself to the small chapel of the hospital and spent the night praying before the crucifix. He then fell asleep and dreamed that Christ had reached out from the cross and touched his diseased leg. On awakening, it was found that his leg had healed completely, with no trace of the cancer.[5]

In the centuries following his canonization, some faithful Roman Catholics and some of other faiths suffering with cancers have implored Saint Peregrine to intercede on their behalf to cure them of their disease. The following is one such novena:

2. Ibid., 163.

3. "Fiber," in *American Heritage Dictionary of the English Language.*

4. Wangerin Jr., *Letters*, 160.

5. Pack, "St. Peregrine," 183–4; cf. Jackson, "Saint Peregrine," 824.

> O great St. Peregrine, you have been called "The Mighty," "The Wonder-Worker," because of the numerous miracles which you have obtained from God for those who have had recourse to you. For so many years you bore in your own flesh this cancerous disease that *destroys the very fibre of our being*, and who had recourse to the source of all grace when the power of man could do no more (emphasis added).[6]

Here, again, the fiber metaphor is employed—only here the fiber is what is basic in us and in all life and is precisely what cancer destroys. Here, too, the science is presciently accurate, for, in its ability to create new environments among healthy cells and to invade healthy tissues, cancer does invade and seek to overcome that fiber of our being. It is for this reason that some faithful have sought aid in their struggle with this disease by turning to saints like Peregrine to join them in their fight. And it is for this reason that the unexpected remission of cancers is sometimes referred in medical literature as "the Peregrine Effect"[7] and that the Lawrence Livermore National Laboratory has developed a program for radiation cancer treatment that it called "PEREGRINE."[8]

While the Novena to Peregrine and, later, Walter Wangerin both connect the term "fiber" to the disease of cancer in nearly opposing ways, each is quite correct in doing so. To say it simply (though complexity still remains): cancer is the very fiber of our being that may destroy the very fiber of our being. It is our own cells—our own life—destroying the life of our cells. In this chapter, we will discuss the ways in which cancer is a disease of cells, the constitutive elements of life that, when they develop in cancerous form, may destroy those very elements. First, we will dive into the science of cellular biology to uncover how it is that "all cells come from cells." We will illustrate how developing cancer cells, too, come from cells. Cancer, then, is not one disease but many diseases constituted by cells originating at different sites in the body; accordingly, we discuss how cancer is one thing in its having a cellular origin and many things in its arising in differing tissue-types. We will explain how all cancerous progressions are dangerous adaptations of normal cellular functions.

---

6. "Prayer to St. Peregrine," lines 1–12.

7. Hoption Cann et al., "Spontaneous Regression."

8. See *Science & Technology Review*, May 1997. The issue was dedicated to the Peregrine program.

Throughout this chapter we will be examining how, given the exquisite order of cellular life, the disorder of cancer comes about. That is, we will be considering how it is that the very fiber of our being is the source for that which may threaten our very being.

Cancer Research: Studies of Humans and Cells

How did cancer research first get its start? While cancer had been identified in patients as a cause of death as early as the time of Hippocrates and probably even before that, research into cancer itself began with the development of the autopsy credited to Giovanni Morgani of Padua, who tried to relate cause of death to underlying changes in the body's pathology. Surgeons later learned that it was worthwhile to try to remove some tumors if they did not invade surrounding normal tissue, and finally after the development of anesthesia in the nineteenth century, cancer operations such as the radical mastectomy and others became more common. All of this work was done with people, but all of these studies were limited because they could report only what could be seen with the unaided eye.

Anton van Leeuwenhoek of Holland (1632–1723) developed a magnifying glass that could be used to count the threads in cloth; he eventually developed approaches for the production of magnifying lenses that he used to construct the first light microscopes. This allowed the examination of microorganisms and cells, the basic units of all multicellular organisms, including humans. With time, it was recognized that each cell is a self-contained unit that carries out processes of metabolism, division, and other essential functions required for life. Microscopic investigation of tumors suggested that cancer tissue and individual cells had a distinct structure from normal cells and also that metastases are actually the spread of cancer cells from one part of the body to another. All of these early studies revealed that cancer was a disease of the cells.

In his 1665 book *Micrographia*, the English scientist Robert Hooke (1635–1703) published some of his many findings garnered through his employment of a then technically advanced microscope. His "Observation XVIII" contains the following remarks on slices of cork: "I could exceedingly plainly perceive it to be all perforated and porous, much like a Honeycomb, but that the pores of it were not regular. . . . These pores, or cells . . . were indeed the first *microscopical* pores I ever saw, and perhaps, that were ever seen."[9] These tiny pores reminded Hooke of the larger rooms or cells in which monks lived apart from one another. During the following two centuries, research into what transpires within these walled-off entities would demonstrate that, in fact, each and every cell, always the basic unit of any life, is an isolated entity, with its own capacity for energy production and metabolism. At the same time it became obvious that, while some cells make up independent individual organisms, many organisms are composed of trillions of cells living in a kind of harmonious community wherein all cells cooperate for the greater good of that community.

As it became clearer that all life is cellular life—that is to say, individual cells either constitute living beings or are, themselves, living beings—questions into the origins of such cellular life arose rapidly. While the speculations of Theodore Schwann (1810–1882) and Johannes Müller (1801–1858) set the stage for developments in cellular theory in the nineteenth century, it was the work of Müller's *Wünderkind* pupil, Rudolf Virchow, that effected significant advances in the study of cells and, thereby, cancer research.[10] "'*Omnis cellulae e cellula*'—All cells [come] from [other] cells," Virchow publicly proclaimed and, though this theory did not originate with him, he became its leading proponent. "All cells from cells"—a simple way to express a profound understanding—is a foundation for cancer research. All these developments subsequently fueled new discoveries about cancer as cellular disorder.

There were two early reports that had significant impact on science's understanding of cancer origins. Bernardino Ramazzini, studying in Italy in 1713, observed that there was an almost total absence of cervical cancer but a high incidence of breast cancer in nuns. He questioned whether these findings were in some way related to their celibate lifestyle. The high incidence of breast cancer was eventually explained by hormones (particularly those associated with pregnancy that protect against this cancer) on one hand, and the low incidence of cervical cancers was found to be related to viruses on the other hand. (Some viruses can lead to cancer development; often sexually transmitted human papilloma virus plays a role in development of cervical cancer). In 1775, Percival Pott of St. Bartholomew's Hospital in London discovered a large incidence of cancer of the scrotums in chimney sweeps; he believed that its occurrence was brought on by soot collecting in the skin folds, bringing forward the concept that a (carcinogenic)

9. Cited by Waggoner, "Robert Hooke."
10. Olson, *Bathsheba's Breast*, 57–58.

compound may cause normal cells to become "transformed" into cancer cells. Eventually, these findings lead to health measures that were aimed at protecting workers from exposure to substances that could increase a worker's risk for development of cancer.

These early studies demonstrated that cancer is a disease of the cells and that environmental factors (perhaps combined with hereditary factors, although this was not understood fully at the time because DNA as the genetic material had not been identified) played a significant role in the induction of cancer.[11]

What is Cancer?

Cancer in the Human Population

Cancer is reported to develop in about 41 percent of Americans, of whom approximately 21 percent will die of the disease. The disease affects everyone, either by having it oneself or having close family and friends who develop it. Overall, in the United States cancer incidences are highest among men compared to women, among African American men and white women compared to all populations, and lowest among Asians of both sexes compared to the entire US population.

It is a mistake to consider cancer as a single disease. Rather, it involves many diseases categorized with the name "cancer" because of the disruption of cell division regulation. Cancer usually starts with a single cell in a single organ that becomes aberrant and develops the ability to invade other organs. Most cancers are named by the organ affected or the cell type in which they originate. For example, breast cancer usually begins in the breast, or melanoma in the skin cells called melanocytes. If each organ and cell type has its own type of cancer, then there are many cancers that can develop. The most common cancer leading to death in the US population is lung cancer and the next are breast cancer for females and prostate cancer for males. The most common type of cancer occurrence in the United States is skin cancer, although there are many forms of skin cancer.

Mammals and many other species (reptiles, fish, some plants, and others) develop cancer as well. Research into animals with cancer often provides information about how we can treat the disease. While mice develop

---

11. For further information about these and other studies that were important in the history of cancer research, see the American Cancer Society website: www.cancer.org.

a large number of cancers on their own, researchers will induce cancers in mice by introducing chemicals or foreign genes in order to provide models for understanding cancer development and therapy in humans.

Pets also develop cancers, and in fact dogs get cancers at about the same rate as humans, with older dogs being more susceptible than younger animals. Sometimes therapies found to be effective in humans were first tested in veterinary clinics to show their value on pets. Cats have slightly lower frequencies of cancer than dogs do.

Cancer in Different Organs

Cancer starts in the body's fundamental unit of life, the cell. Cells and ex-tracellular material make up each organ of the body and carry out most bodily functions in coordination with each other. Cancer undermines this coordination within the body and leads to the dysfunction not only of the organ with the cancer, but often other organs as well, because the body's organs are interdependent.

Overall, cancer is defined as a group of cells that are abnormal in having achieved uncontrolled cell division in a particular location in the body. In other words, the cells are dividing in a way that is no longer regulated like normal cells in the organ or tissue, and this dysregulation leads to the accumulation of abnormal cells in clusters in the body. Any factor regulating normal cell division can become aberrant and lead to the development of cancer.

In recent years, much work and effort has been devoted to the cancer stem cell hypothesis. This model of cancer development is based on the idea that within cancers are certain cells that possess the characteristics associated with normal stem cells: they have the ability to give rise to all cell types. But as we will discuss later, whereas normal stem cells bring about various specialized cells and functional tissues, cancer stem cells give rise to differentiated cancerous cells within tumors. They can be inactive (non-dividing) for long periods of time or they can actively divide and cause tumors to grow. Cancer stem cells may have a pattern of self-renewal that permits them to grow perpetually until destroyed by chemotherapeutic drugs or the host. One interesting component of the cancer stem cell model is that cancer stem cells are particularly resistant to certain therapies such as chemotherapy or radiation therapy. Therefore, when the patient is treated for their cancer with these therapies, the cancer stem cells survive and are able to induce growth of the cancer even after strong treatment regimens, sometimes after several years of "cancer-free" health, i.e., remission.

These cancer stem cells have different properties depending on the tumor of origin and also upon particular genetic changes that occurred in the cells themselves. It appears evident from recent studies that cancer stem cells exist in some, if not all cancers. For example, in some forms of breast cancer, cancer stem cells appear to be highly resistant to therapies and remain dormant in the body for years, permitting the development of a tumor recurrence years after the original tumor was "cured."

Properties of Cancer Cells

What factors regulate cell division? Cell division (i.e., one cell dividing into two) is a complex process involving many pathways with regulatory events occurring at many different points. Each step along the path of cell division depends on the basic molecular processes that occur in all cells: "DNA makes RNA makes protein." This phrase (sometimes called the "central dogma of molecular biology") describes the most fundamental mechanism enabling cells to carry out their functions. Most cells carry DNA (deoxyribonucleic acid), the genetic material, as a source of information for all that that cell can do. Each cell possesses significant resources to maintain its DNA in the form inherited from its progenitor even though this molecule sustains daily damage from different environmental and metabolic sources.

Cellular DNA has to be duplicated before each cell division in order to preserve and pass on cellular functions from one cell to another. The next type of molecule in the "central dogma" scheme is RNA (ribonucleic acid); RNA acts as an intermediate that first transcribes the correct (for the given physiologic circumstances) segments of information contained in the DNA code, and then carries them away from the nucleus into the cytoplasm of the cell. In the cytoplasm most of the RNA(s) are translated into protein(s) in the final step in this process. Proteins carry out most of the functions of the cells, including the regulation of cell division, growth, and development.

Typical steps in the process of cell division are shown in Figure 2. They include three phases: (1) receipt of "divide" signals (and/or "no-division" signals from genes like Rb and p53, which suppress replication of abnormal cells, or cancer); (2) preparations for cell division; and (3) cell division itself.

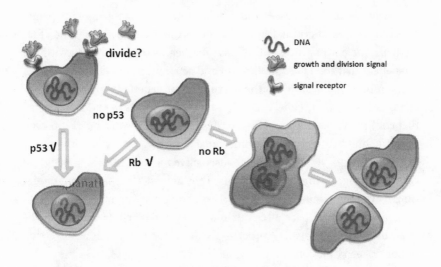

Figure 2: Schematic representation of possible carcinogenesis events
(drawing by Tatjana Paunesku)

The phase of division signal registration (1) might include the following: binding of a growth factor to its receptor on the cell membrane, recognition of this event by other proteins, the phosphorylation (and thus activation) of membrane and cytoplasmic proteins that serves as the signal to divide, and arrival of signal molecules into the nucleus. At the same time, a cell may also receive "no-division" signals either from surrounding cells or its own nucleus. The cell itself may be damaged, too engaged in executing its function in the organism, or unprepared for cell division. When "divide" and "no-division" signals occur in the same cell, the relative intensity of each signal will decide whether the next steps in the process will occur. In many cases "no-division" signals will be stronger and the process stops at this so-called "checkpoint." If the "divide" signal has won, the cell continues onward with cell division.

The phase of preparations for cell division (2) includes the induction of DNA duplication and the new RNA synthesis in the nucleus, the transport of RNAs from the nucleus to the cytoplasm where they are made into numerous proteins: the necessary "everyday" constituents of the cell as well as those proteins specialized for functions associated with the cell division. The cell division itself (3) depends on sequential and well-orchestrated activities of proteins that segregate the available cellular material into two equal parts—two "daughter cells."

Any one of these phases and cellular processes that operate in normal cells can become aberrant, leading to uncontrolled cell division. When that happens, the entire process of cell division begins to malfunction with the final effect that the DNA duplication and separation into daughter cells is done imperfectly, leading to the corruption of genetic information. Each change of the genetic code, called "mutation," increases the odds that a cell that could have been normal diminishes its control over cell division even more. A mutated cell may become capable of division even without any external "divide" signal or become insensitive to "no-division" signals and cease to engage its innate checkpoints. This, in turn, leads to the accumulation of even more mutations. The process of gradual accumulation of mutations, increasing its pace after the loss of regulated cell division, is at the heart of carcinogenesis. The process of cancer development is a subversion of normal cell function.

There are numerous features that make cancer cells different from their neighboring normal cells (Figure 3): (1) cancer cells have an altered appearance under the microscope, being rounded and refractile; (2) they grow on top of one other, ignoring the fact that they are tightly surrounded by neighboring cells (which acts as a strong "no-division" signal for a normal cell); (3) they can proliferate indefinitely with no need for pro-division signals such as growth factors; (4) they can even grow outside of the body in "cell culture" to accumulate a large numbers of cells; (5) they have increased transport of glucose; and (6), if you inject human cancer cells into a mouse that does not have an immune system to attack these cells because they are foreign, a cancer growth will result (something that will not necessarily happen by injecting normal human cells).[12]

12. Flint et al., *Principles of Virology* 2, 201–11.

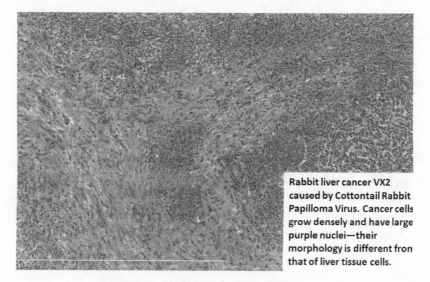

Rabbit liver cancer VX2 caused by Cottontail Rabbit Papilloma Virus. Cancer cells grow densely and have large purple nuclei—their morphology is different from that of liver tissue cells.

Figure 3: Changed morphology of cancer cells compared
to specialized cells that do their tasks

How Do Cancers Grow?

Most models of cancer induction minimally require that a few cellular processes become dysfunctional before a full cancer can form. The multi-step model of cancer formation involves at least three major steps, but most scientists acknowledge that multiple pathways (up to six or seven) usually become dysfunctional before a normal cell can transform into a full-blown malignant cancer cell.

Due to their dysregulated behavior cancer cells often no longer resemble normal cells and to the immune system appear as a "foreign body." Many tumors elicit an immune response in the host that can be used to fight them. One example of a common "self-limiting" disorder is infectious mononucleosis (also called "mono," glandular disease, or the "kissing disease" because of how it is spread). In the United States, most people are infected with the Epstein-Barr virus that causes mono sometime in high school or college. There are a few weeks of discomfort with swollen lymph nodes and flu-like symptoms, and then the disease disappears. Nevertheless, even years later, one can find cells in the peripheral blood of people who have had the disease that retain the ability to divide like cancer cells. Many scientists have studied mono because it behaves like a self-limiting tumor—the cells divide uncontrollably for several weeks, the body mounts an immune response, and this immune response suppresses the progression of the disease.[13] Thus, we can assert that the successful progression of a tumor depends on an evasion of the immune system that the body uses to attack it.

Just as cancer cells in this respect depend on "inactivity" of the remainder of the body, sometimes they also depend on its activity. For example, the tumor itself will not develop its own new blood vessels required for survival from the pool of cancer cells. The cells that develop into new vasculature will be recruited from neighboring healthy cells. Therefore, the interaction between tumor cells and the rest of the body will define the ultimate fate of cancer.

What are the Causes of Cancer?

What types of agents cause cancer? As described above, even in the eighteenth century investigators like Pott of London had determined that chimney soot was involved in the induction of at least some types of cancer. The models describing the induction of cancer include an increasing spectrum of possibilities in recent years. Some of the earliest research involved cancers caused by viruses, mostly in animal systems. Peyton Rous discovered a virus (later named after him—"the Rous sarcoma virus") that caused cancers in chickens and some other birds. Subsequent work by other investigators led to the identification of large numbers of viruses associated with cancer in mice, rats, cats, and other mammalian species. Early investigations in humans turned up very few viruses, but as time progressed, a few viruses were found to be associated with human cancer.

Most notably, human papilloma virus (HPV) was found to be associated with approximately 90 percent of cervical carcionomas and about 50 percent of head and neck tumors; and there is increasing evidence that other cancers may be caused by HPV. Numerous studies have confirmed a role for hepatitis viruses in the development of liver cancer and implicated some HIV-like viruses in human leukemias. In addition to mono, Epstein-Barr virus, a type of herpes virus, has been associated with Burkitt's lymphoma, a lymphatic tumor found more frequently in Africa than other parts of the world. In most cases, cancer-causing viruses deregulate cell

13. Carter, "Infectious Mononucleosis."

division and provide an important step in the multi-step process of cancer formation.

While some human papillomaviruses have been associated recently with the development of cervical carcinoma and some head and neck cancers (and likely other cancers as well), the papilloma virus has been present in mammals for many years. It is interesting to note that in *Animal Qvarvpedia et Reptilia (Terra)* written between 1575 and 1580, Joris Hoefnagel displayed a drawing of different rabbit species; among them was the horned rabbit shown alongside several other rabbit species and presented as a different species of rabbit.[14] In studies done years later, scientists were able to discover that these protrusions on the head of the "horned rabbit" were not actually horns, but were instead giant tumors that were caused by the rabbit papillomavirus, a close relative of the human papillomavirus. The "horned rabbit" was not a new species but rather was a rabbit infected with the virus and bearing a tumor as a result of the virus. This rabbit virus and tumor are still studied in the laboratory today.[15] They are considered important not only because of the virus origin of the tumor (similar to what is found in humans), but also because the resulting tumors when injected into internal organs of the rabbit are similar in structure to what is found in humans.

Some cancers are caused by exposure to chemical substances that cause mutations of the genetic material. Cigarette smoking is one of the most commonly discussed cancer-causing activities because it is preventable. Cigarette smoke has been extensively studied, and over nineteen known cancer-causing chemicals (also called carcinogens) in smoke have been identified. Most of these chemicals are produced by the burning of tobacco and spread with the smoke of a cigarette.

Many other compounds have been discovered to be associated with cancer causation in recent years including asbestos, cadmium, engine exhaust gases, beryllium, and many others. This has led to large-scale governmental efforts to eliminate these substances from occupational and residential environments. Some of these materials had been used in building or manufacturing long before their carcinogenic activity was understood or suspected. Now that their role in cancer induction has been uncovered, the removal of asbestos from buildings or beryllium from manufacturing processes has become imperative. Different food additives (coming from

14. *Wikipedia*, s. v. "Lepus Cornutus."

15. See for example, Lewandowski et al., "Functional Magnetic Resonance Imaging"; Chung et al., "Four-dimensional Transcatheter Intra-arterial Perfusion."

different food preservation approaches such as nitrites, "smoking," or pickling, etc.) have also been implicated as carcinogens and their uses are becoming more limited or better regulated in recent years.

Still other chemical and physical agents that are carcinogenic have been identified and most are regulated by the government. Exposure to radiation has been shown to cause damage to DNA leading to cancer induction, although radiation is relatively weak in comparison to many chemical carcinogens. We are persistently exposed to radiation as part of our natural physical background on the earth, but the government regulates additional human exposure to radiation coming from human-made radiation sources. Regulations for both occupational and non-occupational exposures were developed in order to reduce the numbers of cancers caused by radiation. This is particularly relevant for ionizing radiations (such as x-rays and gamma rays) and exposure to radioactive elements emitting radiation. While high doses of radiation cause radiation toxicities that can lead to death, the major danger from low doses is cancer induction. This has led to much controversy among radiation agencies that find it hard to define exposure dose limits, knowing that even for the low doses, natural and human-made radiation both contribute significantly to the ultimate total exposure.

Exposures to other types of radiation such as ultraviolet light come through sunlight or from tanning beds. While x-rays and gamma rays penetrate the entire body and can induce mutations in internal or external organs, ultraviolet light exposure leads mostly to skin cancer induction. The reason for this is because ultraviolet radiation cannot penetrate beyond the skin with most clothes providing good protection from ultraviolet light mutations in the skin. Low energy radiations (e.g., radiowaves, microwaves, infrared radiation, and visible light) are not associated with cancer causation.

Cellular Processes that Underlie Cancer

In 2000, Hanahan and Weinberg defined six hallmarks of cancer.[16] It is not necessary for each cancer to have all of them, but usually a combination of several of these traits is necessary for successful carcinogenesis. These properties are gradually acquired by cancer cells during the course of development, usually by mutations in the genetic material. The hallmarks *were*:

16. Hanahan and Weinberg, "The Hallmarks of Cancer" (2011).

(1) limitless replicative potential—the ability of cancer cells to continue to divide limitlessly without dying or stopping the process of division; (2) insensitivity to anti-growth signals—the ability of cancer cells to continue growing even when the body is sending out signals to stop dividing; (3) evading a form of cell death called "apoptosis," or programmed cell death—whereas most cells in the body have the ability to "commit suicide" if too many mutations have accumulated too much damage to the genetic material has occurred, in many cancer cells, as indicated in Figure 2, this process is undermined; (4) self-sufficiency in growth signals—the cancer cell no longer requires signals from the body to divide, but rather is able to produce these signals on its own or divide without the signals, so that cellular division is always "turned on" irrespective of the situation; (5) sustained blood vessel growth—cancers develop the ability to recruit and maintain the growth of new blood vessels in order to be supplied with oxygen and nutrients; and, finally, (6) the process of tissue invasion—cancer cells have the ability to invade normal tissue and cause metastases. This invasive process is at the core of the dangerous arsenal of the cancer cell because, if tumor cells were confined only to the tissue of origin and did not interfere with its normal function, the body as a whole would not be threatened by the cancer (death from cancer is caused by the interruption of tissue and organ function). Malignant cancers can invade almost any other tissue, allowing it to spread over the whole body. Just as a crab extends its claws to collect its prey, so does cancer invasively extends itself to new sites to cause death (hence the title "Cancer the Crab").

After Hanahan and Weinberg defined their original hallmarks, new information gained from subsequent cancer research led them to revise their list by proposing two new emerging hallmarks (for a total of eight) and two enabling characteristics that were also features of cancer cells.[17] The idea behind the latter features was that they can tip an already unbalanced cell toward cancer progression and facilitate development of an environment that enhances cancer cell growth. These additional processes are:

> *Emerging Hallmark 1*, deregulating cellular energetics—the dysregulation of energy metabolism and energy utilization by the cell that permits rapid cell division and growth exceeding what one would encounter in a normal cell. (Cancer cells actually need less energy than normal cells in order to function and can reprogram themselves to lower their own energy-making machinery, using

17. Ibid.

less oxygen and requiring lower oxygen consumption in order to function); *Emerging Hallmark 2*, avoiding immune destruction—the development by cancers of some method of evading the body's immune response to fight cancer; *Enabling characteristic 1*, tumor-promoting inflammation—the presence of a large inflammatory response enhances cancer growth in the body. (Exactly how and why this occurs is not fully understood, especially since some forms of inflammation can be useful in fighting the cancer); and *Enabling characteristic 2*, genomic instability and mutation—the ability of cancer cells to cope with and accumulate large numbers of mutations in comparison to neighboring normal cells, with some mutations perpetuating new mutations destabilizing the genome (e.g. through aberrant repair processes, to be discussed in the next chapter), which contributes to further cancer development (i.e., the acquisition of mutations that enable tissue invasion).

Each of these hallmarks and characteristics can develop through several different pathways, in no particular order, and affect different processes in individual cells of a developing cancer. This creates a tremendous variation in the cancers themselves, with very few cancers having exactly the same pathways affected. Due to this variation even the cancers of one single organ are rarely treated with an identical therapy—since each tumor has its own alterations that may be distinct from others, even those of the same organ type.

The Cancer vs. the Cancer Cell

It is important to note that not all tumors are cancerous. A tumor is any type of growth in the body. Often tumors are "benign" in not having the ability to spread beyond their tissue of origin, or in that their cells eventually stop dividing (not having limitless replicative potential). Cancers are types of tumors (or growths) that have several of the hallmark features described above and are usually considered to be "malignant." If left untreated, cancers will take over the body and cause death. All cancers start as single cells, usually undetectable until they reach at least one gram in weight and the diameter of approximately one millimeter. Even at that size, a cancer has one billion cells, many displaying different hallmarks enabling the tumor to continue to expand. When the cancer reaches a total mass of one kg (2.2 lb.), usually the person carrying it cannot survive because the body cannot sustain so much excess mass that is not functional in the body.

Usually the cells comprising a multicellular cancer have considerably more mutations than the original single cell that started the cancer. A process of massive mutation (to be discussed in greater detail in the next chapter) is initiated in the early phases of the cancer, making the final cancer a heterogeneous mass of cells with different genetic mutations and changes in cellular behavior. While one might think that a cluster of cells derived from a single cell would be nearly identical, the fact is that, because cancers develop through uncontrolled cell division and the accumulation of mutations with each step, a developing cancer is a heterogeneous collection of cells with different growth features, dynamics, and interactions. This contributes to some of the difficulties in treating a cancer. While cancer itself is a heterogeneous disease, each individual cancer growth is a collection of cells with hundreds of different mutations supporting each other's continued growth and mutation accumulation.

While the focus of this chapter has been on cancer as a disease of the cells, it is a mistake to think that cancer is only composed of *cancer* cells. There are many other cell types that contribute to the cancer itself: the matrix and basement membrane that provide a site for the cancer to attach to the organ, blood vessels that provide nutrients and supplies to the cancer, immune cells that invade the cancer to fight it, and others. Thus, treatment of the cancer is not only about the cancer cell, but rather about the cancer as a whole with all of its elements.

Cancer Stem Cells

What are stem cells? Stem cells are undeveloped or undifferentiated cells that can become many different types of cells with the proper stimulus. A common example of normal stem cells in the body are cells in the bone marrow that make more new stem cells on one hand or differentiate on the other hand. Through the process of differentiation they may develop into red blood cells (to regulate blood oxygen levels), lymphocytes (to carry out immune functions), platelets (to induce blood clotting), and others. Presence of these stem cells is absolutely necessary for survival. For example, if these cells get killed by a high dose of ionizing radiation, a person so irradiated would die within thirty days after exposure. In such cases, the only hope for the exposed individual is to receive a bone marrow stem cell transplant. Bone marrow transplants have been used for many years and represent a type of stem cell transplant that has been effectively used for many years to treat not only victims of radiation exposures but also to replenish bone marrow in people who had to have their own bone marrow cells killed because of cancer or immune dysfunction.

The bone marrow remains an important source of adult stem cells, but like so many stem cells from adult sources the bone marrow cells have limited utility in what types of cells they can replace. For example, bone marrow can replace hematopoietic (blood cell-forming) cells and serve as a source of blood elements, but it is not likely to be able to replace other cell types in the human body. There is much ongoing work on the use of adult stem cells for treatment of disease; one of the first studies was reported by Kathyjo Jackson and others, and Donald Orlic et al.[18]

While in many cases adult stem cells serve as an important source for experimental research, based on current science, these cells will most likely not be useful against Parkinson's disease, diabetes, or spinal cord injury (as mentioned before—these cells only differentiate into red and white blood cells). For these types of disorders, work with embryonic stem cells is being explored; while these cells are not being used clinically at this time, there is hope that they or additionally modified adult stem cells could be used for replacement of various dysfunctional cells or organ systems in the body.

Cancer stem cells are in some ways similar to normal stem cells because they, too, are precursors of more "differentiated" cells that are in the process of being developed. Most cancer stem cells can give rise to many different cell types in the cancer tissue. Cancer stem cells are different from normal stem cells because they go on to give rise to a tumor rather than to a normal tissue. Cancer stem cells have been identified for many years, but only recently have they been characterized in great detail. Cancer stem cells are tumorigenic, which means that if they are removed from the tumor, they can form another tumor. Not all cells in the tumor have this capacity—very often tumor cells, while they contribute to tumor mass, cannot grow a new tumor on their own. Cancer stem cells can seed a new tumor through the process of self-renewal and differentiation.

Tumors themselves are heterogeneous, and there is currently an understanding that cancer cells within the tumor "evolve" the ability to cooperate with each other as the cancer progresses.[19] The idea that cancers are monolithic and made up of a single type of cells has long been abandoned.

18. Jackson et al., "Regeneration of Ischemic Cardiac Muscle"; Orlic et al., "Bone Marrow Cells."

19. This is discussed in a recent commentary by Chang et al., "Mining the Genomes."

That notion was partially based on overextending the knowledge that cancers are "clonal"—initiated by a single cell. While it is theoretically possible for a cancer to arise from a carcinogen that affects many different cells at one time, most tumors are considered to have developed from a single cell or a single clone. This is called the monoclonal (one-clone) origin of cancer, with all of the cancer cells in a single tumor evolving from a single cell that has gone awry. Each cancer develops from a single cell that acquires new mutations that convey some type of growth advantage to the tumor.

Contemporary understanding of carcinogenesis still acknowledges clonal origins of the initial tumor, but it recognizes a more complex understanding of cancers as the accumulation of many different cell types, and a single cancer being a composite of many different cells and many different diseases.

Another aspect of cancer stem cells that is ambiguous is that on the one hand most cancers cannot be identified as having started from a cancer stem cell (but rather from a normal cell that has acquired a mutation), but on the other that a cancer stem cell can often reconstitute the full tumor, having evolved from the tumor itself. This suggests that one of the dangerous aspects of cancer evolution is the fact that these therapy-resistant, mutated cancer stem cells develop from within the cancer cell mass itself, giving the cancer the opportunity for full regeneration and the escape from therapeutic tools. In other words, while researchers still do not know how to additionally reprogram adult stem cells to be able to make any cell type, many researchers believe that tumors provide a milieu that allows some of the cancer cells to become stem cells that can reconstitute that cancer type on their own. Other explanations of cancer stem cells are also considered, and more about that will be discussed later.

One reason why cancer stem cells are particularly important is that it is thought that they persist following therapy and often leave the primary tumor to seed the metastases. In general, cancer stem cells seem to be resistant to most forms of therapy—chemotherapy, radiation therapy, and other targeted approaches to killing cancer cells.

It is not fully understood why that is so. One idea that is offered as an explanation is that cancer stem cells, similarly to normal stem cells, rarely divide and mostly just "sit and wait" to be needed. This passive existence allows the stem cells to repair almost any type of damage that can be induced by chemotherapeutic drugs, for example. While that is the primary reason why stem cells are able to repair normal tissue damage (e.g., injured liver will regrow due to stem cells), that is also a reason why cancer stem cells will be able to regrow cancer sometimes even many years after the original tumor has been eradicated. The resistance of cancer stem cells to therapy means that they persist even when the remainder of the cancer is shrinking. As such, cancer stem cells limit the curability of the cancer; while they are present in tumors as a small percentage of cells, they remain in the tumor after therapy and thus provide the seeds for a new tumor in the same site or a metastatic tumor in a distant site.

The cancer stem cell model is based on cancer as an "evolutionary process" in the person. One idea that comes out of the stem cell model for cancer suggests that the cancer stem cell can go on to develop into all the different types of tumor cells and thus behave as a true precursor cell. In as second model of cancer stem cells, termed the evolutionary model of cancer (to be distinct from evolution itself), the cancer stem cell is a single cell that mutates and changes to enhance its growth advantage in the host and permit the survival of the tumor. This evolutionary model assumes that mutations that offer a growth advantage for the tumor cell clones will survive and persist in the tumor. Probably each of these two models is correct in some cancers, and even both may be operating in the same cancer, creating a more complicated view of the disease as a whole.

While cancer stem cells were considered to be present in tumors for many years, the first strong evidence to support their existence was reported by a team who identified a specific set of cell surface proteins on leukemic cells, in quantities and concentrations that were characteristic for cancer stem cells only.[20] Following this first report in leukemia, cancer stem cells were found in a large variety of cancers including colon, brain, pancreas, ovary, prostate, breast, and others. The origins of cancer stem cells are controversial and may be different from one type of cancer to another. Different models for the development of cancer cells that have been proposed include mutations that develop in existing normal stem cells, mutants that develop from adult stem cells, and/or mutations that develop in mature cells that give rise to stem cells. Many different physiological and molecular pathways have been shown to be disrupted in cancer stem cells compared to either normal cells or non-stem cancer cells; these pathways are being explored as possible targets for therapeutic agents for cancer treatment.

One of the most usual approaches for cancer research—work with animal models (also discussed in more detail elsewhere)—does not lend

---

20. Bonnet and Dick, "Human Acute Myeloid Leukemia."

itself to fruitful exploration of cancer stem cells. In rodents (which are the primary models for human cancers), work with cancer stem cells is difficult because the lifespan of the mouse is so short that often scientists cannot see the relapse of disease in a mouse treated for cancer. An additional feature that makes therapy of cancer stem cells difficult to monitor therapeutically is the fact that the cancer stem cells make up only a small portion of the entire cancer and therefore cannot be detected well in the total tumor. Therefore, while the total tumor may be shrinking with therapy, the cancer stem cells may remain and render the tumor refractory to the therapy despite the fact that non-stem cancer cells are being destroyed. In essence, the tumor could respond well to therapy, but the surviving cancer stem cells (resistant to the therapy) repopulate the tumor or metastasize, making the tumor difficult to treat.

Summary

Cancer is a disease that starts in a single cell that acquires growth advantages over other cells and divides in an uncontrolled manner. Cancer cells acquire particular traits demarcating them from normal cells that involve the ability to grow without growth signals ("divide signals," Figure 2), the inability to respond to growth inhibitory signals ("no-division signals," Figure 2), the inability to launch a program of cell death (or at least the cessation of cell division) that usually occurs in genetically normal cells, and the ability to promote the growth of blood vessels for their own use independently from general regulation by the body. While cancer starts in a single cell, its daughter cells (its clones) acquire new abnormalities and new "pro-cancer" capabilities with each new cell division, which allow them to spread throughout the body.

There is a mystery of biological being: given the exquisite order of cellular life, why does the disorder of cancer come about? The answer: our cells retain the basic instructions for cell division. Those instructions, the basic drive to divide buried deep within all actively dividing cells, can be unleashed by loss of overarching restraints evolved in multi-celled organisms. Accordingly, the next chapter will focus on genes, which instruct and encode the life of cells. Even with scientific explanations, a mystery remains: the very fiber of our being may the source for the end of our being.

Chapter 2

Chance and Necessity in Life:
Cancer as a Disease of Genes

I n his now classic work, *Chance and Necessity: An Essay on the Natural Philosophy of Modern Biology*, the Nobel Prize-winning molecular biologist Jacque Monod claimed, "pure chance, absolutely free but blind, at the very root of the stupendous edifice of evolution: this [is] central concept of modern biology."[1] From the roots of chance, Monod proposed, biological phenomena developed in conformity to law-like, i.e. necessary, organizing principles. In this chapter, we describe the development of cancer as rooted in the chance and necessity of the molecular activities of genes. In doing so, we reveal how genes provide a simultaneously unifying and highly complex explanation for the causes and the nature of cancers.

Early Theories of Cancer Causation

With the advent of cellular study of cancers in the late nineteenth century, the increase in understanding of contagious diseases, and discovery of heredity, the stage was set to attempt to explain possible causes of cancer as either an outcome of irritation, of contagion, or of heredity. While the exact reasoning behind some of these conjectures about carcinogenesis appears highly implausible, these three perspectives are all actually accurate. With the knowledge we have today we can see that each one of these three

1. Monod, *Chance and Necessity*, 112–13.

paradigms has contributed to a better understanding of cancer as we see it. Moreover, it is highly probable that the science of tomorrow will propose additional possible causes of cancer. It is nevertheless certain that cancer is a disease with a genetic basis. How the genes come to become altered varies, but in its advanced stages cancers carry the burden of multiple mutations.

The concept dominant among researchers and clinicians in the late nineteenth and early twentieth centuries, also ascribed to by much of the general populace, was the one Virchow advanced: "'irritation' in some way provoked not only cancer, but also other ailments for which physicians had no certain explanations."[2] The surmised sources of irritations that brought on cancerous cells were varied and diverse—including jagged teeth, tobacco products, bruises, steel punctures, and sunlight.[3] Evidence that various irritants might induce the disease was presaged by the very accurate observation by Sir Percival Pott (1714–1788) that poorly protected chimney sweeps were prone to scrotal cancers,[4] later confirmed by research findings in the 1920s that "mule spinners"—men who worked at spinning wheels that saturated their crotches with tars and paraffin oils—were also at risk.

To be sure, there were many unresolved issues associated with irritant theory—particularly the length of time between such alleged insults and the manifestation of this disease. However, pragmatic concerns helped the "irritant theory" to achieve and hold high esteem. Its proponents believed that (some) cancers might be prevented by avoiding irritation. In contrast, those proposing alternative explanations for cancer development offered little hope for cancer prevention because its causes, according to them, were beyond human control.[5] Paraphrasing Winston Churchill on democracy, the theory of irritation may have been a very bad one, but to its advocates, all the other theories were so much worse. And just as true democracy may (largely) be a collective delusion, so is the belief in complete comprehension in medicine. Nevertheless, if one sees carcinogens as exposure to cancer causing irritants (see later), this theory has very much merit. Toward the end of the nineteenth century, findings that many diseases such as diphtheria and cholera had infectious origins led to the belief that this was likewise the case with cancer.[6] Additionally, an increased frequency

2. Patterson, *The Dread Disease*, 26.

3. Ibid.; Clow, *Negotiating Disease*, 12–13.

4. Clow, *Negotiating Disease*, 43.

5. Ibid., 49.

6. In Patterson, *The Dread Disease*, 22.

of cancers—whether in specific regions (e.g. towns or streets), or families (such as that of Napoleon Bonaparte)—were offered as evidence of the contagious nature of the disease.[7] Some proponents of contagion theory even thought that many cancers were kinds of venereal disease and, accordingly, attached to their sufferers a similar stigma.[8]

Like those embracing irritation theory, advocates of the contagion theory struggled with its obvious shortcomings—especially the plain fact that cancers did not cluster quite like other contagions. Their best account for this fact was that, just as other contagions do not necessarily produce diseases, so those that might bring about cancer need not always do so. They also argued that, just as symptoms of other contagions that might first be dormant and later become manifest, cancers might first silently smolder and erupt later. We shall see that some of the fundamental premises of contagion theory have their place in contemporary cancer research—while cancer itself is not contagious, some infectious agents may initiate certain cancers.

Just as the notion that contagions caused cancers arose from the awareness that infections caused many diseases, proponents of hereditary origins of cancer relied on the developing conviction that what is transmissible over generations could account for many shared phenomena, desired or undesired—ranging from good skin to addictions, and from genius to antisocial behaviors.[9] Early in the 1800s, hereditary theory of cancer had gained credibility as a result of the work of Henry Earle, a grandson of Percival Pott, who surmised that inherited tendencies brought about more cancers in some chimney sweeps than others—and more among some family clusters of chimney sweeps than others. However, it was the resurgence in the early twentieth century of Mendel's theory (dating from the mid-1800s) of genes as hidden elements handed on across generations that provided the intellectual fuel for theories of the hereditary origins of cancer. From this perspective, the "dread disease" was not the result of chance contagions or random irritants, but rather the end product of law-like genetic regularities.

What is interesting about these early models of cancer is that isolated aspects of each of them are known to be true today. We know that some cancers are initiated or accelerated by "irritants"; for example smoking has

7. Clow, *Negotiating Disease*, 5.
8. Patterson, *The Dread Disease*, 23.
9. Ibid., 38.

been shown to play a major role in development of lung cancers as well as cancers of throat, mouth, nasal cavity, esophagus, stomach, pancreas, kidney, bladder, and cervix. Regarding the contagion model, recent studies have demonstrated that some forms of stomach cancer develop following ulcers caused by infection with the bacterium *Heliobacter pylori*. This type of bacterium resides in the stomachs of some people under specific acidic conditions. We also know that some viruses (such as human papilloma virus, discussed below) initiate the development of cancers. Finally, heredity is firmly established as a primary cause in some cancers, particularly childhood cancers (also discussed below). The early investigators were on the right track; their stories were just incomplete! Much more importantly, these researchers have apparently insisted on a single point of view— "unified" explanations—while ignoring the context of their complete contemporary research. While scientists today accept the possibility that their explanations are (still) incomplete, most of them try to encompass as much pertinent data as possible when they develop theories. With regard to cancer, we know that each cancer cell carries multiple mutations. The routes by which these mutations accumulate are too many to be explained in detail here or even for all to be mentioned. However, several of the best-known sources of (cancer-causing) mutations are listed, including those of the three historically "controversial" points of view.

Cancer Research: Cancer as a Disease of the Genetic Material

The German zoologist Theodor Boveri, working in 1902, is credited with being the first to provide evidence to support the idea that cancer is a disease involving chromosomes. In 1902, scientists still did not know that DNA was the genetic material, but it was believed that chromosomes carried the genetic material and were large units of inheritance that were transmitted from one generation to the next. Ultimately, the credit for that discovery fell to an American evolutionary biologist and geneticist named Thomas Hunt Morgan. He received the Nobel prize for first demonstrating that chromosomes are important in heredity.

The chromosomes, we now know, are large structures that can contain thousands of genes (the X chromosome for example is estimated to have 1,529 genes in humans). Boveri was able to manipulate chromosomes and observe how chromosomal division (which is always preceding cellular division) can become aberrant leading to uncontrolled cellular division. He proposed that this event of scrambling of chromosomes could come from a variety of different insults to the cell, including radiation, viruses, chemicals, and other similar injuries.

Thus, even though Boveri was not considered to be the one who proved that chromosomes are carriers of heredity (although he was fully convinced of that fact because of the results of his research), and even though he did not dream that the DNA is the critical chromosomal component with hereditary information, he was the first one to see that many different types of cellular injuries can lead to chromosomal aberrations. Subsequently, the idea that cancer is a disease of the DNA was furthered by studies of virally induced cancers where cancer could be caused by the introduction of a single virus into the DNA of the host cell. These studies led to the uncovering of dominant and recessive oncogenes (discussed below) and the modern theory of cancer as a disease of the DNA.

Genotoxic Damage

Cancer has often been considered to be a disease that primarily affects DNA; while changes in protein or RNA are not passed on the daughter cells when the cell divides, changes in the DNA are. Thus, treatments like heat that predominantly cause changes to proteins are not usually carcinogenic because those changes will not be passed on to the next generation of cells. Cells that have sustained heat damage will either be repaired or die before cell division can begin.

Most agents that cause cancer (mentioned above as carcinogens) do so by damaging the genetic material, the DNA. Because this damage is a type of genetic toxicity, these agents are also called "genotoxic agents" or mutagens. Very few carcinogens have been identified that are not genotoxic, but alter cell growth control nonetheless. These include agents like hormones and some organic compounds. In most cases, the mechanism of carcinogenesis by non-genotoxic agents is poorly understood. For the most part, while these agents do not cause DNA damage directly, "natural" mutations occur and accumulate because of the rapid proliferation of cells. Most carcinogens are also genotoxic, which means that they induce DNA damage that leads to mutations.

When mutations arise in the DNA, a number of changes can occur: new proteins with slight differences from the normal protein can be made that never existed in the body previously; proteins can be truncated or deleted; and protein amount or location in the cell can become dysregulated so that it no longer supports normal cellular function. All of these changes can contribute to unlimited cell division characteristic of cancer cells. As discussed in the previous chapter, cancers arise from a single cell that proliferates and changes with each cell division as the cancer grows in the individual.

A recent census of genes involved in cancer identified 291 genes in the human genome which, when mutated, lead to cancer development. Although this number has been revised several times since, the salient point is that more than 1 percent of all the genes in the human genome can play a role in cancer. Of these mutated genes, 90 percent are found in the somatic cells of the body (which includes any cell except eggs and sperm), 20 percent can be inherited (they occur in eggs and sperm as well), and 10 percent fit into either group.[10] The next sections examine the specific categories into which these cancer-associated genes subdivide.

Dominant Oncogenes

In the previous chapter, we noted that some cancers can be caused by viruses. As a matter of fact, a majority of the early cancer research discoveries dealt with viruses identified in rodents, chickens, and other experimental models. It was often found that the DNA of the virus carries a specific segment that transformed normal cells into cancer cells. Early investigators interested in oncology (literally "study of tumors") called these pieces of DNA "oncogenes" because these viral genes caused cancer when introduced into the appropriate cells. The Rous sarcoma virus mentioned in the previous chapter was found to carry an oncogene called *src* that caused sarcomas in chickens. After this first discovery, over thirty oncogenes were found in other viruses specific for mice, rats, cats, chicken, and monkeys.

What was fascinating about these oncogene DNA sequences was that similar, but not identical, DNA sequences were found in the genomes of all mammals (including humans). Further investigation showed that the oncogene DNA sequence in the virus genome was often a mutated or truncated version of the related sequence in the genome of the host. While the non-mutated, full-length sequence of these genes did not cause cancer (every normal cell of every healthy mammal carries these genes), modification

10. Futreal et al., "A Census."

of the gene by mutations or acquisition of a mutated gene through viral exposure led to cancer. This was the first hint that mutations in specific normal genes (later called "proto-oncogenes" because they could give rise to oncogenes if mutated) could contribute to the development of cancer.

While normal genes were called "proto-oncogenes" it soon became clear that the role for these genes is to regulate cell growth and development. These genes are not ticking time bombs waiting to cause cancer; their normal function underlies necessary growth of tissues and organs. Only if mutated or altered, when they cause aberrant control of growth and cell division, do proto-oncogenes become oncogenes that could initiate development of cancer.

Another interesting aspect to these proto-oncogene sequences was that, in at least some examples, the genes themselves were not altered at all; rather what was altered was the *regulation* of the gene. While the gene was normal and the protein it produced was correct in shape and function, the quantity or timing of the protein production was abnormal. In these cases, a perfectly normal gene could now be turned on to very high levels in a cell (sometimes instead of five copies of the normal protein the cell had 500 copies) and this was enough to cause the cell to be a step ahead on the road toward carcinogenesis. These gene regulation changes also involved mutations, not in the protein-coding region of the gene, but rather in the portion of the gene that controlled the turning off and on of gene activity. Thus, an oncogene can also be a gene for a protein expressed at abnormally high levels in the cell and causing cellular division changes associated with cancer induction.

The simplest to be identified, and therefore the first to be discovered, were so-called "dominant oncogenes." These cancer-inducing genes behaved like dominant genes typically do in the genome—i.e., when either one of the two copies of the gene was mutated, the cells became altered, a step closer to becoming cancer cells. These dominant mutations were considered to be "gain of function," which means that the mutant gene had a new function that could not be ascribed to the original normal proto-oncogene.[11]

An example of a dominant oncogene would be a protein that normally needs to encounter a "pro-growth signal" (e.g., one of the growth factor receptor proteins needs to bind a growth factor) before it sends to a cell a signal to divide. The dominant mutant form of the receptor no longer needs

11. See Brown and Hinds, "Tumor Suppressor Genes."

40

to be bound to the growth factor; it sends the signal to the cell to divide all the time, regardless of the presence and binding of the growth factor. This is a new function that was not part of the original functioning of the growth factor receptor in normal cells.

An interesting finding about these dominant oncogenes was that they could be found in mutant form in a large variety of different cancers from different cell types and tissue types in different organs. The dominant onco-genes showed little if any cell-type specificity in their cancer-causing ability. All the dominant oncogenes fall into the category of genes associated with cancer development in somatic cells in the body (all cells other than egg and sperm cells), and no inherited forms of dominant oncogenes have been identified in mammals. This means that no person inherits a dominant on-cogene mutation from their parents—all mutations in dominant oncogenes are acquired during the lifespan of the person either through exposure to genotoxic chemicals, viruses, or some other combination of insults.

Dominant oncogenes were found to be associated with a variety of different types of genetic changes in human cancers. Changes in chromo-some structure associated with leukemias and some cancers that are found in tissues are commonly associated with changes in particular oncogenes that caused protein production at very high levels. In fact, this is the most common mutation among the known cancer genes that have been identi-fied to date. Mini-chromosome like structures have been found in some cancer cells that contained thousands of extra copies of dominant onco-genes, leading to the production of excess protein from that gene. Small mutations are found in some oncogenes that caused the mutant protein product to have increased in activity compared to its normal counterpart. Almost every type of mutation that can alter the production, stability, or activity of an oncogene has been found in one example or another. Most oncogenes identified to date fit into the category of dominant oncogenes.

Recessive Oncogenes

It soon became clear that dominant oncogenes did not explain the entire story of cancer causation, and investigators began to look at other mecha-nisms involved in cancer induction. Of particular interest were those can-cers that appeared to be inherited in a familial pattern where there was some association between genetics inherited from parent(s) and cancer development, but no oncogene could be found to be involved. Investigators began examining families with high incidences of particular types of cancers to determine which genetic component could be observed to be cancer associated.

One of the first such examples was studies about the disease "retinoblastoma," a rare tumor of the eye most frequently found in familial form in children diagnosed most frequently before the age of four. In familial retinoblastoma, a dominant inheritance pattern was found for the disease (which means that 50 percent of the offspring will develop the disease), yet no known oncogene that was mutated could be found in these patients. It was then proposed that perhaps the disease involved the inheritance of one recessive gene followed by the mutation of the other normal copy of the gene.[12] Recessive genes are never expressed unless their genetic counterparts (most genes exist in pairs) are also mutated or lost through genetic deletion. According to this model, the person inherited one mutant copy of the retinoblastoma mutant gene (called Rb) from one parent, and one normal copy from the other parent. Then, during the course of eye development, a mutation in a single cell occurs, eliminating the remaining normal Rb gene copy and giving rise to the tumor growth starting with such a single cell. Subsequent studies of this particular model proved it to be correct.

Studies of heritable cancer susceptibilities led to the discovery of recessive oncogenes, oncogenes involved in cancer causation only when *both* copies of the gene are lost by deletion or lose their function because they have mutated. These genes are also called tumor suppressor genes because as long as one functional (non-mutated) copy of the gene was present, the tumor did not develop—the tumor development is *suppressed* through the activity of these genes.

There were several features that made tumor suppressor genes distinct from the dominant oncogenes described above. They were "loss of function" genes: the cell had to lose the function of these genes totally in order to become a step closer toward becoming a cancer. In addition, tumor suppressor genes were discovered because they were specifically inherited from parent to child and their mutation gave rise to very specific tumors. Rb gene mutations, in general, did not give rise to other tumors except retinoblastoma. This tissue specificity for the tumor suppressor genes is still poorly understood today even after decades of study.

12. Knudson, "Mutation and Cancer."

After Rb was discovered, several other tumor suppressor genes were discovered because of the inherited nature of particular tumors. Among these were the genes called: WT (gene associated with familial Wilms' tumor), APC (associated with familial adenomatous polyposis coli), E-CAD (gene connected with familial gastric cancer), MEN1 (associated with multiple endocrine neoplasia), and more. First to be discovered among tumor suppressor genes were those whose absence led to development of tumors in children. However, as studies were expanded, genes associated with tumors in adults were also identified.

As mentioned above, loss of tumor suppressor genes generally leads to cancers of specific tissues and organs, so tumor suppressor mutations associated with adult cancers were discovered as specific cancer types "running in families." For example, multiple endocrine neoplasia can be found in children, but the most common age at diagnosis is thirty-eight. One exception to the "tissue specificity rule" is the tumor suppressor gene p53; this gene was found to be mutant or dysfunctional in close to 90 percent of cancers. Its absence is causatively associated with the development of all types of cancers including breast, lung, lymphoma, soft tissue sarcomas, and more.

A recent example of a tumor suppressor gene that has received much public attention is the Brca1 gene that is associated with a higher risk for development of breast cancer in some women. The gene encodes a protein important in DNA repair, i.e., in maintaining the integrity of the genetic material in the face of damage to the DNA. The Brca1 protein is important in several different DNA repair pathways, but one copy of the normal gene is sufficient in order to allow for normal repair in mammalian cells. However, when one copy of this gene is defective, then there is a chance that the other will become mutated as well. Those cells with two mutant Brca1 genes have inefficient or inappropriate repair and accumulate mutations every time the DNA is damaged and needs repair. Thus, otherwise slow processes of mutation accumulation become more rapid in people with Brca1 deficiency, with eventual initiation of cancer being a likely consequence of those mutations. The curious thing about the Brca1 (and also Brca2) gene is that scientists still do not understand why a defect in the gene with such a universal role in DNA repair should predominantly give rise to tumors of the breast in both women and men (or breast and ovaries for Brca2).[13] Both the Brca1 (and Brca2) proteins are used by all cells of the body for DNA

13. The role of Brca1 and 2 in breast cancer has been well studied in the literature. One of the first reports was King et al., "Breast and Ovarian Cancer Risks."

repair. A better understanding of the tissue specificity of cancer development caused by tumor suppressor genes is needed.

Understanding that tumor suppressor genes actually produce proteins that somehow suppress cancer development caused great excitement in biomedical research circles. There was great interest in exploring these genes to determine whether they could be exploited as cancer therapies. Like dominant oncogenes, these genes also regulated cell cycle control and development. For example, the normal Rb gene produces one of the proteins that act as "checkpoint" proteins (Figure 2) and regulate progression of cell division.

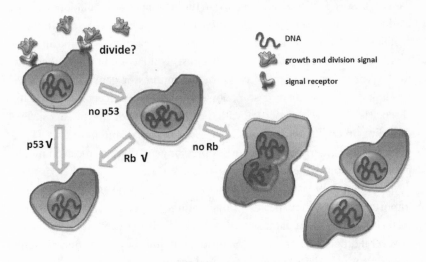

Figure 2: Schematic representation of possible carcinogenesis events
(drawing by Tatjana Paunesku)

In non-human mammals, viruses were found to carry dominant oncogenes that have been incorporated in the viral genetic material. While these genes do not harm the virus, they lead to cancer development in the host organism. In humans, however, few viruses were found to carry dominant oncogenes. Instead, human cancer-causing viruses more often carry genes for proteins that deactivate tumor suppressor proteins through protein-protein interactions. Thus, in humans, virally caused cancers have an organ-specific expression pattern that is similar to cancer type specificity associated with tumor suppressor gene mutations.

For example, the human papilloma virus (HPV) is known to be associated primarily with the development of cervical carcinoma. How does HPV lead to cancer development? When HPV infects cervical cells, it produces proteins that inactivate the tumor suppressor protein, p53. Cells deprived of the benefits of functional p53 presence do not repair DNA damage properly and undergo deregulated cellular division. Thus, infection with the virus transforms an otherwise non-mutated cell into a cell which divides uncontrollably even in the presence of plenty of p53 protein in the cell. It is reported that over 90 percent of cervical carcinomas have normal genomic sequences for the p53 gene, but the p53 protein activity is absent because of the presence of the viral proteins that inactivate it.

Several other viruses are known to inactivate tumor suppressor gene proteins, including simian virus 40 (SV40), adenovirus, polyomavirus, several members of the herpesvirus family, and the Epstein-Barr virus. The mechanism of enhanced cancer development due to the activity of viral proteins that inactivate tumor suppressor proteins is a common mechanism of the viral promotion of cancer in humans, although viruses are not considered a major cause of cancer in the human population.

Other Gene-Related Changes Associated with Cancer

Telomeres

All organisms that have linear (not circular) chromosomes have short repeated DNA sequences at the chromosome ends that are called telomeres (from *telos*, which means "end"). These short sequences protect the ends of the DNA from unraveling or fusing with other chromosomes, functioning something like the aglet (hard casing) at the end of a shoelace. The telomere length varies with species, being shorter in yeast, for example, than in humans. In human stem cells and embryonic cells telomeres are long, while their length is shortened with every cell division in all other cell types. As the person grows and develops through cell divisions and the cells become specialized for different final functions in the body, their telomere length becomes shorter and shorter. When the telomere length becomes too short, any future cell division is prevented, until the cell eventually dies.

Cancer cells are unusual because, regardless of their telomere length at the time of transformation into a cancer cell, they undergo limitless cell divisions. This is possible because cancer cells activate an enzyme that never permits the telomere length to become so short that cell death is induced. This is another way in which cancer cells are immortalized and continue to grow forever. Telomere shortening is a mechanism that cells use to sense how old they are and determine whether the ends of chromosomes are sufficiently stable to last through more rounds of cell division or not. For cancer cells, though, this "sensing" mechanism (one of the important "no-division signals") is turned off, and cell death or the cessation of cell division for cancer cells is thwarted by yet another mechanism.

Epigenetic Changes

Epigenetic changes are changes to the activities of the genome that do not include a change in the actual DNA sequence information. There are many steps in the regulation as to whether a particular gene is turned on (made into protein) or not. Most epigenetic changes involve chemical changes either to the DNA itself (without affecting the genetic information it carries) or to the proteins bound to the DNA. Recently, researchers have also identified RNA molecules that do not themselves serve as templates for protein production but rather regulate ability of other RNAs to be transcribed. As some of these targeted RNA molecules are transcribed into dominant oncogenes and tumor suppressor proteins, these regulating RNAs can augment (and perhaps even initiate) a process of carcinogenesis. Most epigenetic changes are complex and can have different effects in cancers of different cell or organ lineages.

There are a variety of changes that appear to be "epigenetic," which means that they take place "above" or "around the genome" and not necessarily effect an actual change in the base sequence of the DNA. "Epigenetics" is a broad term used to define all changes that influence the expression of the genome but are not in themselves genetic. The most commonly studied epigenetic modification is gene methylation, the presence of a methyl group ($-CH_3$) on the DNA. Usually, this methyl group is added to the DNA on particular nucleotide residues (usually cytosine [C] residues that have a neighboring guanine [G] residue). Methylation usually "silences" a gene, makes it not to be used by the particular cell even though the gene is present and even expressed in other cells in the same person.

The process of methylation provides one method for the cell to control gene expression and to "turn off" at the same time many genes that are present in the DNA and prevent them from being made into proteins. Genes are often methylated not only in their coding region but also in the region that regulates binding of protein factors that initiate the process of gene expression. There are a large number of cancer-associated gene suppression events that are regulated by methylation. The genes silenced in cancer include some DNA repair genes, some tumor suppressor genes, cell cycle regulatory genes, and more.

The genes normally silenced in differentiated, functional cells, on the other hand, are often activated in cancer cells through demethylation. The entire genome of a cancer cell has much less methylation than a normal cell; many people have hypothesized that this global epigenetic change may promote genomic instability and chromosomal abnormalities.

Another wide-ranging epigenetic change that is associated with cancer is modification of proteins called *histones*. Histones bind to the DNA and regulate its "openness," the degree to which it is ready for access to factors that initiate and regulate DNA replication (necessary for chromosome duplication prior to cell division) and DNA transcription into RNAs (which constitutes gene expression). When certain histone proteins are modified they can regulate the level of gene expression and even DNA replication. In cancer cells, there is a decrease in the acetylation of histones, i.e. a decrease in the presence of acetyl groups on the histone proteins. Usually, this decrease in acetylation can result in silencing genes that are tumor suppressor genes, effectively turning them off so that the cancer can progress.

MicroRNAs provide another level of epigenetic change in cancer cells. MicroRNAs (or miRs) are small and very stable RNAs that often regulate many genes at the same time by binding to the RNAs produced by gene transcription and preventing them, through different means, from being translated into proteins. If one or several suppressor genes are being targeted by a specific miR or a group of miRs, then there will be a new step forward in the progression of the cancer.

Some anti-cancer therapies have been developed that target these epigenetic changes. Some drugs prevent methylation and permit anti-cancer genes to be turned on that would otherwise be silent. These hypomethylating drugs have been found to be useful in preventing the progression of a pre-leukemic state (called myelodysplastic syndrome) to a full leukemia. Another category of drugs called histone deacetylase (HDAC) inhibitors have gone through many clinical trials for use in a variety of tumors. These drugs prevent the removal of acetyl groups from histones and thus allows for gene reactivation even after the cancer has put in motion mechanisms that will inhibit gene expression. These types of epigenetic therapeutics are often used in combination with chemotherapy and immunotherapy for treatment of the patient. Finally, researchers are currently investigating many different types of anti-miR molecules. This research is made difficult by the fact that miR molecules are very stable and produced in large quantities in cancer cells.

Mutations and Cancer

Cancer is a disease caused by dysregulation of many genes. The initial steps in the process may be very simple, leading to a single gene being dysregulated, but as the cancer develops (evolves) in the individual, new mutations accumulate with each cell division. Each new mutation in any of the genes mentioned above constitutes another step in the cancer progression. In the multistage model of cancer development, the first step usually involves a genetic change that allows for the cell to escape from the normal control mechanisms regulating its activity as a part of the tissue. As a cell progresses from this pre-cancerous phase to a progenitor cell that will divide into all cells that make a cancer, a large number of mutations in dominant oncogenes and tumor suppressor genes accumulate, until the cancer reaches a stage of genomic instability.

This phase in cancer development is characterized by the rapid accumulation of a large number of mutations within the genome. Order and type of mutations that emerge are different in each cell in the course development of any specific cancer, and, while all the cancers are initiated with a single or a few genetic changes, over the course of the lifetime of the cancer, its cells acquire a multitude of different additional and unique mutations. This means that even though it begins with a single cell, the advanced cancer is composed of a disparate population of cells with many different specific mutations.

An average cancer of the breast or colon can have sixty or seventy mutations that lead to the production of altered proteins that are beneficial for furthering cancer development. Compare these mutations in cancer cells to the frequency of mutations we find in normal cells: ordinarily there are 0.35 mutations in comparing all sequences that make protein from parent to child; this means there are a total of seventy new mutations per generation in all the genes that make up the human body. Cancers have a huge mutation rate compared to normal cells.

What is the cause of this high mutation rate in cancer cells compared to normal cells? Much research has shown at least in some cases defects in

DNA repair arise due to mutations in the genes that code for proteins that execute DNA repair. There is a battery of 100–200 proteins responsible for maintaining the integrity (or intact-ness) of the human genome, carrying out the surveillance function and repairing errors that might occur in genomic DNA. These errors may result from errors during DNA replication, endogenous DNA damage, or damage from exposure of genetic material of cells to exogenous chemical and physical sources of DNA damage (such as carcinogens or irradiation). Mutations in some DNA repair proteins can lead to the development of a "mutator" function in the cell, permitting mutations to remain uncorrected in the genome. Cells that have one or more dysfunctional DNA repair proteins can acquire this type of mutation function, which leads to increased genomic instability and the accumulation of mutations in cancer cells. There are more than forty inherited human repair gene mutations that increase a person's risk for developing cancer. Some of these cause the repair functions to be less efficient than usual, while others inhibit particular repair pathways altogether.

In fact, the search for elusive human DNA repair proteins was facilitated by the idea that cancer would be expected to result in those people that had abnormalities in their ability to repair DNA damage. It had been known for many years that agents that cause damage to DNA also lead to the induction of cancer; it was not known how this link occurred. Scientists speculated that if a patient developed a higher rate of cancer than normal people following exposure to DNA-damaging agents such as sunlight or ionizing radiation, then perhaps these patients had an inborn defect in a DNA repair protein. These patients were identified and studied, and indeed, it was found that they had inborn mutations in particular genes. When the proteins coded for by these genes were studied, they were found to be important in pathways associated with the repair of DNA damage following exposure to various environmental DNA-damaging agents.

Some of these DNA damaging agents were found in the natural environment that all organisms on earth receive exposure to—sunlight, background radiation from space, chemicals in plants, and others. This resulted in the identification of a large number of DNA repair proteins and multiple pathways of DNA repair for different types of damage that an organism might encounter in its lifetime.[14] This led to the idea that cells had evolved mechanisms to handle DNA damage from our natural environment; over time, this model has been shown to be true.

14. See for example Lehnert, ed., *Biomolecular Action*.

All organisms that live on earth, from the smallest bacteria to humans, have evolved DNA repair pathways that are used to handle DNA damage that results from living in our natural environment on earth. What is interesting is that the repair mechanisms in different organisms have many similarities. The genes encoding proteins that handle DNA damage from ultraviolet rays found in sunlight are similar in bacteria and humans, and the multi-protein regulatory pathways to handle this damage are also similar and related.

Moreover, recent studies have shown that DNA damage comes not only from our environment but also from metabolic activity of our own cells. Endogenous oxidative damage to our DNA can cause as many as 50,000 DNA lesions per cell per day. In the healthy person, there is a balance between DNA damage and repair. However, when cancer (or some other disease associated with a high cell division rate) develops, the balance is tipped against repair leading to the increased accumulation of mutations in cells. Many people try to supplement their diets with antioxidants (green tea, blueberries, and other similar foods) in an effort to reduce the accumulation of innate oxidative damage in cells.

It is interesting to note that cancer is not the only disease having a high mutation frequency. Large numbers of mutations have also been found in some neurologic diseases including Lou Gehrig's disease (amyotropic lateral sclerosis), Alzheimer's disease, and others, although it is not clear whether these mutations contribute to disease progression in the same way as they do in cancer.

Cancer and Inheritance

While many genes have been associated with cancer development (and probably many more are yet to be discovered in the coming years), and while cancer is a disease that begins with the DNA, it is clear that not all forms of cancer are inherited. In fact, the majority of people who go on to develop cancer do not have a genetic susceptibility for it. Previously we saw that mutations in tumor suppressor genes can be inherited as one copy of the gene and lead to a higher chance of developing a cancer as a second mutation if the counterpart gene is acquired. These cases, nevertheless, are rare when one examines all cancer cases.

Twin studies have been done investigating the genetic component that might contribute to cancer. The idea behind these analyses is that identical twins with identical genomes should have similar cancers developing at similar ages and in similar locations in the body if there is a genetic component to the disease. Fraternal twins, with a much smaller degree of genetic similarity, serve as the control group in these studies. These research efforts have shown that there is no concordance for specific cancers when identical twins are compared with fraternal twins.[15] This suggests that, while there are some known genetic factors that contribute to the development of cancer, environmental factors play a more important role in cancer genesis.

Cancer and Cancer Treatments

While tumor suppressor genes were found as causes of childhood cancers, many predominantly pediatric cancers appear to have only a minimal inherited component. In such cases, youth of the organism (longer telomeres, ongoing growth, etc.) often confounds the treatment prognosis additionally, while fear of long-term damage to the child limits the spectra of possible anticancer treatment tools.

For example, the most common cancer in childhood that occurs outside the brain—neuroblastoma—in only 1–2 percent of cases has an apparent hereditary component. This poorly understood cancer can change from a highly malignant state to take on a completely benign cellular appearance, yet 20–50 percent of patients do not respond to therapy at all, and even some who do respond initially go on to relapse and eventually succumb to the disease. Despite the name, this tumor is rarely found in the brain; instead, it starts in nervous system tissue located in other parts of the body, often nerve tissue in the adrenal gland that sits on top of the kidney. The cancer is very hard to treat because there are many different types of neuroblastomas with many different mutations that have been found in different patients. Thus, the treatment regimen that is effective for one neuroblastoma is often not successful for others.

In adults, while more drastic therapies can be used, many cancer types still represent a challenge that is often beyond the hope of curative treatment. On the other hand, cancers successfully treated may be associated with additional problems. A second cancer can develop in patients (and especially young patients) who have responded appropriately to the treatment for a primary cancer. Sometimes years later these individuals develop a second cancer that is different in type from the original. There are many

15. Risch, "The Genetic Epidemiology of Cancer."

reasons why secondary cancers develop, and not all are clearly understood. These cancers are often studied in the adult survivors of childhood cancers.[16] For example, many young girls who were treated with radiotherapy for the lymphoma called Hodgkin's disease, between twenty and thirty years later develop a secondary breast cancer in the radiation field; this suggests that the secondary cancer developed as a result of the radiation exposure treatment for the primary cancer. Some chemotherapy-induced cancers appear even earlier, often within the first ten years after exposure and often as a type of leukemia.

In addition, there may be a genetic component to these secondary cancers since a person could have a genetic susceptibility associated with the development of the first cancer. Cancer survivors are urged to have yearly evaluations for secondary cancers since this is a risk associated with most therapies. This is discussed in more detail in the next chapter.

Summary

Cancer is characterized by a high DNA mutation frequency. Normal cells in the body usually have a very low mutation frequency due to safeguards preventing the accumulation of mutations in somatic cells. Cancer is a multi-stage process in which a single normal cell acquires the ability to proliferate outside of the context of the normal tissue. And, as the cancer grows through cell division, its cells acquire more and more mutations, giving the cancer as a whole a growth advantage. Cancers can have as many as between sixty and seventy mutations supportive of cancer development compared to normal cells.

In this chapter, we have learned that genes are the information repository and the instructional base for a system that smoothly flows along, usually. When that flow is disrupted, cancers may develop. Understanding the nature and processes of genes provides a fruitful understanding of the nature of cancer—fruitful in its revelation of just how complicated cancer is. That complexity resides not only in what genes are and do, but also in how genetic processes are driven by evolutionary forces of chance and necessity. In the next chapter will examine the ways in which these forces are at work in the evolutionary disease of cancer.

16. The Children's Oncology Group has been studying secondary cancers that develop in adults who were treated as children for cancers. See www.childrensoncologygroup. org.

Chapter 3

Hallmarks of Oncological Development: Cancer as a Disease of Evolution

Cancer Research: Cancer as a Disease of Evolution

C ancer is an evolutionary disease in two different ways. First, it evolves in the patient over time and changes with the changing environment of the body. Cells of the metastasis are different from the cells of the original cancer; and, as the body makes its own chemicals to attack the cancer, the cancer evolves to evade them. This dynamic process has been recognized only recently and it is at present shaping much of the ongoing research in the field. The facts that cancer evolves in the person and that some of the principles of evolutionary adaptation and selection occur in cancers are applied to how investigators think about cancer. It is certain that this will have an increasingly more important role in future cancer research. The second way in which cancer is a disease of evolution is one of the main focal points for this book—the fact that cancer itself is a disease that is inevitable because of human evolution. Biological understanding of this thesis is expanded upon below.

What is Evolution?

This chapter focuses on relating cancer and evolution, but requires both a preliminary definition of "evolution" and an examination of the limitations involved in conjoining the topics of cancer and evolution.

"Biological evolution" is defined as *descent with modification*. This definition includes both "small-scale" evolution (such as changes in the frequency of a particular gene within a population from one generation to the next) and "large-scale" evolution (such as the descent of different species from a common ancestor over many generations). Charles Darwin, a British naturalist who explained that species develop over time and developed from a common origin, first proposed evolution as a biological theory. His two most important works are *On the Origin of Species* (first published in 1859) and *The Descent of Man, and Selection in Relation to Sex* (published in 1871).[1] The major tenets proposed by Darwin and accepted by the mainstream scientific community to this day were: (1) that there is a common ancestry for all life on earth; (2) that species develop through variations in form (now known to be the result of inheritable mutations); and (3) that nature "selects" variations and drives speciation.

Evolution was originally presented as a scientific theory, a logically self-consistent model describing the behavior of a natural phenomenon originating and supported by observable facts. Like all scientific theories (such as the theory of gravity, the theory of relativity, etc.), evolutionary theory is formulated, developed, and evaluated according to the scientific method. Often in everyday language, people equate the word "theory" with "speculation" or "conjecture." In scientific practice, however, the word *theory* acquires a very specific meaning—it is a model of the world (or some portion of it) from which falsifiable hypotheses can be generated and verified (or not) through empirical observation of facts. In this way, the concepts of "theory" and "fact" are not opposed to one another, but rather exist in a reciprocal relationship.

The dictionary definition of evolution describes it in a broad sense as a process of change accompanied by some selection process, but biological evolution itself is much more limited in definition. Biological evolution has a "direction" that depends on the genetic pool of the population that lives in a certain environment and the changes in that environment acting upon

---

1. See Darwin, *On the Origin of Species*; *The Descent of Man*.

the population through natural selection. Douglas J. Futuyma, in his book *Evolutionary Biology*, makes the following distinction:

> In the broadest sense, evolution is merely change, and so is all-pervasive; galaxies, languages, and political systems all evolve. Biological evolution . . . is change in the properties of populations of organisms that transcend the lifetime of a single individual. The ontogeny of an individual is not considered evolution; individual organisms do not evolve. The changes in populations that are considered evolutionary are those that are inheritable via the genetic material from one generation to the next. Biological evolution may be slight or substantial; it embraces everything from slight changes in the proportion of different alleles within a population (such as those determining blood types) to the successive alteration that led from the earliest protoorganism to snails, bees, giraffes, and dandelions.[2]

Biological evolution, then, does not act upon individuals, but rather upon groups of individuals called "populations."[3] The fate of individuals can be affected by their traits, but individuals do not undergo biological evolution. While changes we undergo in life may perhaps be called "personal evolution," they do not relate to the biological evolution of our species. A natural unit enacting biological evolution is the population. In terms of biological evolution, a population represents a collection of genes and genotypes (all the specific forms of genes that each specific person carries), and the evolution of the population in time can be expressed as a change in the frequency of certain genes and genotypes over the same period of time.

Mutations in the DNA (changes in the hereditary material of life) are the drivers of evolution. Normal cells in the body, as noted in the previous chapter, are remarkably stable with respect to their DNA sequence and use multiple mechanisms in order to maintain their genetic information without changes. Mechanisms to protect the DNA of somatic cells of the body from developing mutations with high frequency have evolved; and DNA repair pathways and high fidelity DNA replication mechanisms have evolved to serve this function. Nevertheless, if mutations never occurred in eggs or sperm cells, no new genetic information could be passed on to offspring, so that evolution could not occur. While this new information may in some circumstances be detrimental to the individual that carries

2. Futuyma, *Evolutionary Biology*, 751.

3. Smith and Szathmáry, *The Origins of Life*; Wilson, *Darwin's Cathedral*; Woloschak, *Beauty and Unity in Creation*.

it, changes in the environment modulate the force and direction of natural selection. Occasionally, new genetic information is better suited for a new environment and natural selection ensures that the new genetic material spreads in the population. In this way natural selection drives evolution, using genetic variations as its fodder. In each case organisms with the best survival advantage multiply, while others with poorer adaptation to the environment are reduced in numbers.

Mutations are random, (generationally) transmissible changes to the genetic material. They can be beneficial, neutral, or harmful to the organism that carries them in a given environment. Not all mutations are relevant to evolution, and some mutations can occur that have no (immediate) impact on evolution and persist in the genetic pool of the population until they become harmful, useful, or vanish by chance.

Mutations occur in all cells of the body; there is no biological mechanism that would prevent mutations in one cell type and allow them in another. Mutations in somatic cells (cancers form in somatic cells) are not passed on to offspring and therefore are not drivers of evolution. Mutations in germline cells are rare and mutated genes accumulate in a population slowly across generations. Nevertheless, the low frequency of mutation accumulation is in the right balance with relatively slow changes in direction of natural selection, leading to gradual biological evolution. Too high a frequency of mutations in each generation would contribute to an unstable genome that could not support life.

Chance and Necessity

In biology, the ideas of chance and necessity are often used to describe events that happen randomly (chance) or under defined and precise conditions (necessity). Arthur Peacocke, to whom we will return in chapter 6, is one of the scholars who described the differences of chance and necessity in evolution.[4] However, chance and necessity are phenomena well understood in all life sciences. Perhaps the easiest way to understand them is through some examples afforded by radiation exposure.

Following exposure to low doses of radiation, we see few immediate apparent consequences in people or animals. We do know, however, that such low doses of radiation can lead to an increased incidence of cancer,

---

4. See Peacocke, "Chance and Necessity in the Life-Game." The importance of Peacocke's contribution is reviewed in Woloschak, "Chance and Necessity."

and the lower the dose the less likely the chance of cancer developing. This is a chance phenomenon that depends on whether the radiation damages the cell, the DNA, or an oncogene. The chances for each one of these events occurring can be calculated only when many cells are considered at the same time. For any single cell, exact prediction of the damage caused by radiation is not predictable.

Non-random (often called "deterministic") effects of radiation occur in the same way and under precise and predictable conditions; thus they are considered to occur by necessity. Cancer and mutations are considered to happen by chance, but other tissue responses to radiation (e.g. development of cataracts or reddening of the skin) occur at defined doses and exposure conditions. Non-random effects occur predictably and can be anticipated. For example, if a person receives a given dose of radiation (2Gy) in one short exposure given directly to the unshielded eye, one can predict that the person will develop a cataract within six months to two years after the exposure. This and other deterministic effects occur only at high doses and are believed to be caused by tissue damage and do not occur by chance.

Any attempt to relate evolution and cancer has to be founded on the fact that both evolution and cancer induction depend on mutations, which in turn occur by chance. Some of the same mechanisms involved in mutation generation, therefore, will be responsible for both processes, even though the scope and effect of mutations in these two cases is different. Those mutations that are a part of the process of evolution affect any one of the genes in the complete genetic code of germ cells, while mutations associated with cancer are generally found in a relatively limited set of genes, primarily in somatic cells. Also, most mutations associated with evolution have no immediate bearing for the individual in which the mutation occurred; rather, they become a part of population's genetic heritage to be selected or lost over time through natural selection. Most mutations causing cancer, on the other hand, have drastic short-term effects on their bearer and originator.

Evolution and Cancer

Many processes described in the previous chapters define changes in the genetic material that occur in cancer cells in contrast to normal cells, and it was noted that a large number of the different changes in the genetic material of somatic cells accompany the development of cancer. Some types of genetic changes, albeit in a smaller numbers per each single cell, occur in eggs and sperm (also called germ cells) and become genetic material of the next generation and thus can lead to evolution. So, while cancer-free survival for a single individual is best secured by high fidelity DNA duplication and accurate corrections of genetic information after DNA damage, evolution depends upon occasional mistakes in these processes (Figure 4).

Actually, the processes of DNA duplication and correction have been "honed in" by evolution to be, in a limited degree, error prone in all cells including, therefore, both germ and somatic cells. This error-prone process ensures that some mutations will be incorporated into the genetic material, in some cases the genetic material of germ cells (possibly contributing to evolution and much more rarely to cancer in the next generation) and in some cases that of somatic cells (possibly contributing to cancer). In germ cells, the mutations are caused by the same agents that cause mutations in somatic cells—radiation, viruses, chemicals, and others.

New mutations (shown as change in line color of melanoma cells) accumulate in majority of melanoma cells as the cancer grows and cells divide. These mutations further speed up cell division and cancer growth.

A single new mutation is "fixed" in the grand-daughter. All of her children will carry a new version of hair color gene (which may or may not provide them with the survival advantage.

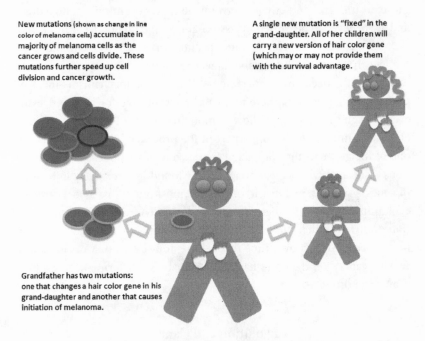

Grandfather has two mutations: one that changes a hair color gene in his grand-daughter and another that causes initiation of melanoma.

Figure 4: Schematic diagram of mutation accumulation in cancer vs. future generations. Figure was drawn by Tatjana Paunesku.

As natural selection removes detrimental genetic traits from populations, one could imagine that genes supporting error-prone DNA duplication and repair processes would have been uprooted from the genome if they caused more harm than benefit to the species. The fact that the capacity for introducing errors into genetic information is firmly fixed as one of the traits of every species of living organisms on earth means that the long-term survival of any species requires that capacity. Therefore, even if some species (hypothetically) did evolve to a state of error-free DNA duplication and repair, such species would have become extinct as soon as any serious change in their environment occurred. No earthly environment is changeless, and, therefore, the force of natural selection is always changing its direction. If a population of organisms of the same species successfully inhabits one geographic region, environmental changes in that region may lead to local extinction unless the population as a whole has sufficient genetic variability to produce individuals suited to survive in the new environment.

Both selection and evolution "work" on populations of organisms, but cancers do no not participate in this process. As mentioned before, cancer cells become separated and different from functional cells in the organism that harbors them; they never produce germ cells, only more cancer cells. Changes that occur in cancer cells in contrast to normal cells are not incorporated into germ cells and, therefore, do not contribute genetic material to a population's genetic pool. The oncogenes that are activated and tumor suppressor genes that are inactivated all die when the cancer dies. How, then, does cancer relate to evolution? It is primarily through the process of cancer formation and, hence, cancer is in part the price that we must pay for our evolution (at least for evolution into humans).

Humans and all other species have evolved processes that repair our genetic material when damaged, correct our DNA when duplicated improperly, and work to keep the DNA integrity and genetic information intact. Nevertheless, as previously mentioned, complete changelessness of the DNA information pool would result in species extinction. Changes in environment that occur over time modulate the pressure of natural selection and "new" traits (resulting from mutations of existing genetic material affecting sometimes exact function of proteins or regulation of their synthesis) may eventually become advantageous in "new" (changed) surroundings. Biological evolution is the change in the genetic information pool of a population of individuals in response to its changing external situation. The only way for new versions of genes to appear in the genetic pool is through mutations in germ cells, and, therefore, evolution demands that some aspects of the process of DNA maintenance be imperfect so that mutations can occur in the germline cells, allowing for at least a low frequency of mutated new versions of genes to appear in the genetic pool with a new generation. There is no inherent "goodness" or "badness" to any individual mutation. It is only through natural selection that a mutation will be preserved or discarded from the gene pool of the population. However, this small deficiency in the system of DNA maintenance means that some mutations will also occur at very low frequency in somatic cells, making a first step toward development of a cancer.

Most models of DNA repair pathways suggest that, if humans (or any other multicellular species) could live long enough, they would all eventually develop cancer.[5] This means then that cancer as a disease is natural for humans in the sense that it is a condition that is a carry-over from our evolutionary biology. In a sense the development of cancer may be inevitable in the absence of other causes of death.

Some people believed that cancer was a disease of the modern era ushered in by pollution, automobile exhaust fumes, coal-burning smoke, and other components of a modern industrial (or post-industrial) culture. Others have argued that it is only the relatively short life-span of our ancestors that caused most to die before they had a chance to develop cancer. Hippocrates (460–370 BCE) first used the word *carcinos* to diagnose cancers he found in his patients. Some ancient fossils of humans from 3000–4000 years ago have been identified showing that cancer was found in ancient populations.[6] Most scientists consider that, while cancer is an old disease that has been around probably since the existence of the human species, the reason why we are seeing it in patients with increased frequency is because we have eliminated many other causes of death, so that now people can live long enough to develop cancer. Before 1945 and the discovery of antibiotics, average life expectancy was fifty years, much lower than it is now because catching pneumonia or some other infectious disease would be enough to kill the person. Following the discovery of antibiotics, life expectancy has increased by thirty years, leading to cancer as one of the major causes of death.

5. See Alberts et al., *Molecular Biology of the Cell*, ch. 20.

6. Several reports have documented this: Jarus, "Egyptian Mummy"; see also "Researchers Find Cancer."

An aspect of evolution important to remember is that it operates on the level of species as a whole and, consequently, fitness of any individual beyond the reproductive years has little bearing on the genetic makeup of the next generation. For a species with a long (non-reproductive) childhood like humans, the ideal situation for maximal contribution of new genetic material to future generations would be for each generation to live forty to fifty years, rear numerous progeny, and then die, thereby freeing those resources for the next generation. This would mean that human bodies would have to be active and functional only for forty or so years and that no effects of selection pressure could be exerted by people beyond that age.

On the other hand, while this "model" would apply to a species made of unconnected individuals, there are indications that it does not fully apply to humans. For example, a number of scientists have argued that menopause is an overall benefit to the population because it allows women to contribute their assistance, knowledge, and skills to other group members, thus enhancing group fitness.[7] Still others have shown that human evolution may be distinct from that of most other species because there is a dependence on grandparents for greater support of the offspring.[8] This model remains controversial among evolutionary biologists and anthropologists.

Cancer as an Evolutionary Process

Biological evolution in its proper sense can be associated only with the process of natural selection occurring on the level of populations in natural surroundings. Nevertheless, in a broad sense, the word *evolution* can be applied to any change accompanied by some selection process, although the mechanisms may not be identical to those found in a natural selection process. The successful development of cancer in a person has been frequently compared to evolution because, as the cancer cells mutate, a selection process promotes or removes some of the cancer cells from the cell pool. Those cells that can grow best and fastest quickly constitute the greatest bulk of the tumor. Some people call this process "somatic evolution."

The cancer starts with a single cell that has some type of growth advantage in the body. As cell division progresses, the daughter cells acquire large numbers of mutations randomly, and those cells with the best growth advantage over their "sibling cells" become the most numerous in the

7. Campbell, *Human Evolution*; Williams, "Pleitropy."
8. O'Connell et al., "Grandmothering."

population of cancer cells. There is even a selection process for those cells that can grow best at sites distant from the primary tumor body. In fact, some mutations have been identified that are specific for metastasis and best allow for a tumor to grow in a particular metastatic environment.

Among the challenges that cancer must overcome in the body are the immune mechanisms of the host that are designed to kill the cancer. Many cancers develop mechanisms to fight off the immune response by, for example, altering their membrane proteins so that the cancer is no longer recognized as "non-self," as a foreign invader.

Another common type of evolutionary change in cancer is the development of drug resistance. When chemotherapeutic drugs are first given to the patient, they are in most cases somewhat effective against the cancer, damaging the rapidly proliferating cancer cells so much that they die or stop dividing. Nevertheless, as long as some of the cancer cells survive the treatments and the cancer continues to grow in the presence of the drugs, cells that harbor mutations providing drug resistance begin to grow better than their drug-sensitive counterparts. In one type of drug resistance, the cancer produces very high quantities of a protein on the cell membrane that shuttles any small molecule (such as chemotherapeutic drugs) out of the cell as soon as it enters the cell. This, too, is a type of evolutionary process that is ongoing in the cancer cell population.

The thing to keep in mind is that selection again acts on all the cells present (population of cells), and it selects those that already have the mutations advantageous under the given circumstances. This selection process is much like natural selection in that the cancer cell best able to survive drug treatment is the one that survives in the host (regardless of how many cancer cells die due to mutations that do not support growth under the given circumstances).

There are many groups studying cancer as an evolutionary process because there are so many parallels to what one finds in the biological evolution of species. In cancer, there is a selection for cell populations that carry mutations giving them a survival advantage over other cells. In biological evolution, there is a selection for individuals among the population of a species that have acquired from their predecessors the mutations giving them a survival advantage over others individuals. In both cases, there are competitions for nutrients and other factors that are present in limited supply. In addition, in both cases, mutations are the drivers in the selection process.

It needs to be mentioned that developing the cancer itself is a survival disadvantage to the individual because the person prematurely may die from it. While the cancer develops in the individual, in the end, the presence of cancer itself leads to its own death by killing the organism serving as its host. The cancer is similar to a parasitic relationship, growing in the person at the expense of their health. The cancer steals away nutrients, energy, minerals, and other bodily needs that deprive normal cells of the host of these materials. If left unstopped the cancer takes over the person's body until the body cannot sustain it.

Transmissible Cancers that Evolve

One unusual type of cancer that is transmitted from one animal to another is the canine transmissible venereal tumor (CTVT). This tumor is passed from one dog to another as a cell or group of cells, predominantly through copulation, although other routes of touching among dogs (licking, biting, sniffing, etc.) have also been suggested to play a role. The cancer cells are a transmissible agent that arose over 11,000 years ago in a founder canid and has been transmitted (as a sexually transmitted disease) from dog to dog ever since. This cancer is the longest surviving cancer.

Recent studies have sequenced the genomes of CTVT from a variety of different dogs and their findings suggest that the tumors arose long ago, but underwent changes about 500 years ago when humans began to breed dogs for specific traits. While the CTVT samples themselves are remarkably similar in having a stable makeup from one tumor to the next, they have acquired a huge number of mutations during the course of their evolution. The genome of the standard CTVT has 1.9 million mutations, orders of magnitude higher than the few thousand mutations found in most other non-transmissible (and therefore short-lived) tumors. It is difficult to discern all of the factors that may contribute to this high mutation rate over the millennia, but about 42 percent of the mutations have a particular signature that is found in cancers caused by exposure to the ultraviolet radiation found in sunlight.

The CTVT is a remarkable example of tumor evolution that has occurred not only in the life time of a single dog, but over the life-spans of dogs for 11,000 years.[9] This is the longest continuously living cancer that

9. Murchison et al., "Transmissible Dog Cancer Genome"; Thomas et al., "Extensive Conservation."

is known, and the evidence for evolution of tumors is clearly evident from this example.

A similar tumor has been found on the faces of Tasmanian devils. This, too, is a transmissible cancer, but the mutation frequency of this tumor is lower, with 20,000 mutations compared to normal cells from the animal. It is not certain how long this tumor has been in Tasmanian devil populations.

Evolution of Cancer Cells in the Test Tube

Much work has shown that normal cells can develop into cancer cells in the test tube given the right conditions and that the process involves a selective process similar to evolution, in which the cells best accustomed to the test tube grow the best and take over the entire culture. When fetal cells are removed from a hamster and placed in culture, they grow normally for a few generations. After about ten passages in culture (or ten changes of the medium), they begin to look more like cancer cells than normal cells with many of the characteristic features of cancer cells mentioned previously. These cells then hit a "crisis point" where they do not grow well, being almost unable to divide; during this period normal cells die off through a normal process of aging. Most models of cell culture growth suggest that normal cells go through cell division only a limited number of times. Slowly, after five to ten more passages in culture, a clone (or perhaps a few clones) of cancer cells emerges from the original normal cells. These clones have acquired a few mutations in dominant oncogenes and recessive tumor suppressor genes that made them closer to becoming a cancer. This development is an adaptation for growth in the test tube representing a selection process for those cells that are immortal in specific cell culture conditions. In fact, if they remain in culture long enough, they will develop all the characteristics of cancer cells so that, if one were to inject them into a mouse without an immune system, they would become fully grown cancers.

Cancer research has been highly dependent on the use of cancer cells cultured from patients and the normal cells that have acquired the features of cancer cells during their time in culture. The first cultured cancer cells that were immortalized when grown in culture were the HeLa cells derived from and named after a cervical carcinoma patient, Henrietta Lacks, who died from her cancer in 1951. Much has been written about these first cancer cells that revolutionized cancer research.[10] The development of this first line of cancer cells that could be grown outside of the body allowed for all the studies of genes associated with cancer, *in vitro* testing of drugs that might be effective against cancer, and much more. The cells were interesting because they were immortal in the tissue culture plate and could be grown very rapidly. They were also the first cell line ever to be cloned.

HeLa cells are the most studied cancer cells in the world and the DNA sequence of these cells is available in GenBank.[11] In fact, it was controversial when the DNA sequence from HeLa cells was released; for most cell lines, the identities of the patients are not known, but for HeLa cells, because they were the first established cell line, the identities and the family of the patient became known to the general public. In addition, because Henrietta Lacks did not give permission for the cells from her biopsy to be used for research purposes, all of the work developing her cell line and experiments done with it were without her permission.

The release of sequence information on Henrietta Lacks's cells also gave information on the (partial) DNA sequence of her children, something that is considered unethical under most conditions. For that reason, the sequence was taken down from the National Institutes of Health (NIH) website and investigators could not use the information gained from the extensive sequence work done on the HeLa genome. Following a series of negotiations between NIH and the Lacks family, eventually an agreement was reached and the sequence information was re-posted on the website and made available to cancer researchers worldwide.[12]

Since the development of the HeLa cell line decades ago, numerous cell lines from other types of cancers have been established in culture. There are limitations to working with cells in culture in that they do not always share identical responses to drugs and other agents as the cancer in the whole organism. For that reason, human tumors are often studied when injected into mice that have had their immune system eliminated

10. See for example Skloot, *The Immortal Life*. Skloot notes that in 2009 over 60,000 papers had been published about HeLa cells with the number increasing at a rate of approximately 300 new papers per month.

11. GenBank is a website supported by the National Institutes of Health in the US that makes gene sequences freely available as an annotated collection of all publicly available DNA sequences; www.ncbi.nim/nih.gov/genbank/. The HeLa cell genome was first published in the following paper: Landry et al., "The Genomic and Transcriptomic Landscape."

12. Callaway, "NIH Director"; see also "NIH, Lacks Family Reach Understanding."

so that the human cancer cells are not rejected as foreign by the mice. The use of these human tumor models in mice is a major way in which studies of efficacy of different drugs and other agents are tested and experiments are conducted to understand how cancers spread, how they invade other tissues, etc.

Genomic Instability in Cancers

Genomic instability or genome instability is a situation where a large number of mutations "spontaneously" occur in cells of a particular lineage. Genomic instability can be an outcome of anti-cancer treatments (chemotherapy or radiation), but it is also very often innate to cancer cells, as well as some neurologic diseases such as amyotrophic lateral sclerosis (or Lou Gehrig's disease). In normal cells, great cellular energy is expended in efforts to maintain genomic stability, with the outcome that chromosomes and chromosome numbers remain very stable. In normal cells, the mutation rate is approximately one protein change per generation.[13] In contrast, the cancer cell genome is not under the same stringent regulation with regard to chromosomal division and DNA repair. It is this genomic instability of the cancer cell that permits the cancer to "evolve" in the host.

Were the cancer genome stable, genetic changes associated with the rapid evolution of cancer cells in the body would not be possible. In contrast to biological evolution of species, which takes place over millennia because mutations are passed on only in the germ cells and because of the extreme stability of the genome of most organisms, cancer "evolution" inside an organism can take place rapidly because the cancer genome is so remarkably unstable. Going back to normal cells, it is worth noting that DNA repair mechanisms, which prevent genomic instability, are highly conserved among species. Some of the same processes that occur in bacteria relate to those found in mammalian cells; this attests to how important these processes are for survival of species on earth. All life on earth is exposed to a variety of different environmental insults, thus all of life developed and retained mechanisms to cope with those insults, including DNA repair. In fact, it is known that the rate and accuracy of DNA repair processes has an influence on the evolution of organisms.

The genomic instability of cancer cells is often expressed as a "systems-wide" instability. Genetic mutations under any circumstances occur

13. Keightley, "Rates and Fitness Consequences."

randomly, not only in those regions of the genome that code for proteins but also in non-coding DNA. When studies have been done on cancer cells comparing their gene sequences to normal cells of the same type, as many as 333,000 small mutations have been identified.[14] It has been reported by some studies that as much as 1.5 percent of the entire genome of a cancer cell in a fully developed tumor is mutated compared to its normal counterpart.

What causes the genomic instability of cancer cells? In most cases it is caused by an initial damage to genes that are important in repairing the DNA when it has been damaged or when the cell has undergone a large number of replications in a short time (which is also one of the features of cancer cells). DNA repair is mediated by a series of cellular pathways that are complex and permit the cells to respond to damage that might be encountered during everyday exposures—background radiation, ultraviolet radiation from sunlight, normal damage during cell division. Some pathways for DNA repair are essential for life and in their absence life cannot exist.

For example, when mice were created without some of the genes for DNA repair, the damage gradually accumulated in the bases in the DNA of embryonic cells and these mice died as embryos. There are some cases of repair mechanisms that are required less regularly, e.g., some people can survive until teenage years even with the repair defect, if they are supported by hospital environment and sheltered from exposure to radiation damage.

Patients with a rare disease called ataxia-telangietasia (AT) are not able to repair breaks of the double-stranded DNA helix. While individuals with this disorder might survive into their teens, their DNA repair sensitivity is so extreme that patients with the disorder cannot survive exposure even to a low-dose chest x-ray. People with AT often go on to die prematurely from leukemia or some solid cancer in their late teens or early twenties. The absence of the ability to repair their DNA properly leads to an innate genomic instability that contributes to the development of cancer.

While global defects in DNA repair are rare in the human population, they are almost all universally associated with an increased propensity to develop cancer because of the link between failure to maintain genomic integrity and cancer induction. Other well-known DNA repair disorders include xeroderma pigmentosum (sensitivity to ultraviolet radiation),

---

14. The example of melanoma cells, which has such a large variation, was reported by Berger et al., "Melanoma Genome Sequencing."

Fanconi's anemia (sensitivity to DNA cross-linking agents), and severe combined immunodeficiency (sensitivity to ionizing radiation).

In people who have normal DNA repair capacity, permanent increase in genomic instability can occur because of a single mutation in a single somatic cell that leads to a DNA repair abnormality in that cell alone. This creates a cell clone that is not able to repair DNA properly and can accumulate mutations rapidly. In this example, a single gene mutation in a DNA repair gene sets the cell up to have the ability to accumulate mutations and therefore becomes genomically unstable. This situation of genomic instability in a single clone of cells sets up the further situation where mutations of all sorts can accumulate with each cell division and lead the mutated daughter cells to "evolve" into a full-blown cancer. While the cancer begins from a single cell, the cells that it divides into during so-called clonal expansion are genetically diverse.

This genetic variability, where individual cancer cells have different mutations and survive in different circumstances, makes cancer such a resilient disease. The metastatic cells often have different mutations than the original parent tumor. The tumor evolves to have the features that are optimal for the particular environment where the cells are growing.[15] There are now at least thirty-four different inherited mutations in DNA repair genes that have been shown to relate to the induction of cancer.

Some diseases associated with failed DNA repair also lead to premature aging. Among these are Bloom syndrome and Werner syndrome, both of which involve defects in a protein that unwinds the DNA and is important in both DNA replication and repair. Most individuals with one of these disorders also die of cancer at a young age, usually before age twenty-five. Because these individuals also display symptoms of premature aging, many researchers have linked cancer, DNA damage, and aging. In addition to cancer, natural aging appears to involve a loss of fidelity of DNA repair and replication.

The DNA damage model of aging has suggested that aging is a consequence of, on one hand, accumulation of naturally occurring damage in the genetic material, coming from natural sources; and on the other hand gradual slackening of damage repair by the cells of an aging organism. Some of these natural sources of DNA damage would include sunlight, radiation in the environment, reactive oxygen species that arise during normal

---

15. Much of the information presented here can be found in textbooks of cell biology, for example Lodish et al., *Molecular Cell Biology*.

biological processes, chemical reactions, and others. There is of course a relationship between aging and cancer, with cancer being more common in persons who are older. It is also possible that the normal loss of fidelity of DNA repair and replication may contribute to the cancer induction that is associated with aging.

One of the interesting observations that relate cancer and aging is the finding that caloric restriction in animal models of DNA repair disorders often increases the longevity of the organisms as well as their health. The mechanisms by which restriction of calorie intake can influence DNA repair and enhance the lifespan of the organism are not clearly understood, however. Some researchers have pointed to a nutrient-sensing pathway and activity of mitochondria as playing an important role in regulation of genomic stability through DNA repair. It is interesting to note that caloric restriction has not only been shown to increase lifespan but also to decrease a variety of different diseases in mice, including arthritis, heart disease, and others.[16]

Somatic Evolution and Cancer

The first idea that cancer was a disease that may evolve in the body came from the work of Boveri,[17] who argued that aberrations of chromosomes lead to cellular deformation and cancer and that the changed chromosomes were inherited from one cancer cell to another. When it became understood, more than fifty years later, that DNA is the key molecule of inheritance, scientists were able to connect specific genetic mutations with particular chromosomal abnormalities, and the genetic basis of cancer became clearer. It also became known that chromosomal changes progressed/accumulated with the development of the tumor, and each of these changes was associated with particular mutations. The process of cancer evolution could be identified as a series of genetic mutations that accumulated with time and that lead to a growth advantage for the cancer cells compared to the normal cells in the body.

As has been noted several times in this book, cancer develops through an "evolutionary" process that selects for cells with the best growth advantage in particular locations in the body. The process of mutation accumulation is much faster than that in evolution of species, which occurs naturally over generations of organisms. This is predominantly because cancers

16. Spindler, "Rapid and Reversible Induction."
17. This work was described by Manchester, "Theodor Boveri."

develop the ability to mutate at a very rapid rate, as described above in the section on genomic instability. Moreover, cross-generational evolution of species depends on occasional mutations of germ cells—sperm and egg cells that each bring, at the moment of fertilization, each comprising one complete half of the entire DNA content of the future organism. While "evolution" of cancer begins with any single cell of the body, most often it is a somatic (non-germ) cell, mutating at high rate.

The process of somatic evolution of the cancer in addition to rapid mutation acquisition involves selection, which explains to some extent why cancers are so difficult to cure. While natural selection pushes evolution of species in directions best suited for survival of the whole species (often at the expense of specific individuals), effects of selection on cancer lead to cancers best suited for survival at the expense of the host.

There are three main features that are considered important for selection in cancer. First, there must be variations in the population of cells that make the tumor, which separate them from the rest of the organism and each other, i.e., the cancer must be a combination of different mutant cells with genetic and non-genetic features that distinguish them from normal cells. Secondly, the variation must be heritable, transferred from the mutated cell to its daughter cells through the process of cell division or cellular reproduction. Thirdly, the variation must affect survival and reproductive fitness of the cancer cell for the particular environment where it is located in the body. As is noted above, diverting usual cell division and cell death processes is part of the development of oncogenesis.

Within the body, tumor cells compete with normal cells for nutrients (particularly glucose), oxygen, and even space. Therefore, mutant cells that compete successfully for these limiting materials will divide more, and grow more than the surrounding non-mutant normal cells. One important example of this is glucose metabolism. While most cells are able to produce their own (chemical) energy that allows them to fulfill their functions, all of them also have the ability to take up glucose from the bloodstream and use it as an efficient source of energy when needed. This glucose uptake depends on activity of glucose receptor proteins located on the cell membrane that recognize the glucose molecule and transfer it from the extracellular to the intracellular space.

Cancer cells often acquire mutations that increase the number of glucose receptor proteins on the cell's surface, this in turn permits cancer cells to have higher glucose uptake than normal cells. In this way, cancer cells can often successfully compete for sugars, taking up more than normal cells and even depriving normal cells of their nutrients. In fact, some of the diagnostic tests established to detect cancer cells use this capacity of cancer cells to identify them in the body. The imaging technique positron-emission tomography or PET scan, when coupled with injection of radio-traced glucose molecules, provides a 3D map of sites of glucose uptake in the body. PET scans can reveal where cancer cells are because their uptake of glucose is so much higher than the surrounding normal cells.

Competition for space, on the other hand, involves local and regional expansion of the tumor, as well as metastasis. Because cell motion through the body requires many different cellular activities, governed by multiple genes, cancer cells that are capable of invasion are those that have acquired many mutations. Because the mutation process, even in cancer cells, is gradual, early tumors with fewer mutations are generally not able to sepa-rate from the rest of the tumor and begin progression through the body. That is the primary reason why an accepted way to evaluate the stage or grade of solid tumors is based on how far they have spread from the pri-mary tumor site. The more advanced the tumor the more spread it will be because it will have acquired more mutations. By the same token, the more mutations (of any type) a tumor has the better it will be able to withstand any new selection pressure, including anti-cancer therapies.

Ultimately in a cancer, the cells that are best able to compete for ma-terials and space divide and expand. The process where one single cell with ideal features for maximal use of its environment divides and grows to make up a majority of the tumor cells is called "clonal expansion," the con-tinued growth of a single clone of cells. As the environment changes (either locally or because the cancer cell has metastasized and left the tumor), new mutations from the pool of mutations generated due to genomic instability are selected for. This leads to a seeming paradox that although cancers arise from a single cell, the final tumor and tumor spread harbor vast amounts of genetic heterogeneity.

It should be noted that while genetic heterogeneity of cancer allows for selection of the cancer cell that is most fit for particular environmental circumstances (including coping with anti-cancer therapies), cancer ulti-mately leads to the death of the host. Therefore, at the level of the popula-tion (and the entire species) and from the standpoint of natural selection, capacity to develop cancers is a negative trait, especially if cancer-bearing individuals are "culled" from the population before reproductive maturity.

Therefore, natural selection on the level of the species selects for genes and processes that suppress tumor development. Among the mechanisms naturally evolved to prevent cancer occurrence are immune responses, activities of tumor suppressor genes, anti-tumor proteins made by the body, and more. Therefore, while the cancer itself is "evolving" in the body, the population as a whole has evolved processes that fight cancer.

One aspect of the evolutionary model of cancer that makes therapies so difficult to achieve is the fact that each cancer is always unique because it has its own unique set of mutations in each one of the tumor cells. While the tumor is mutating rapidly, those with mutations that do not support an individual cell's survival will be eliminated from the tumor quickly, while those mutations that permit enhanced growth will be positively selected for in the population of cancer cells. Because this process of mutation induction is random, the genetic makeup of two tumors in two individuals will be distinct. In fact, the genetic makeup of two tumors that arose independently in the same person will be distinct. This has lead to a very challenging situation for development of therapeutic approaches; trying to develop a single tactic to destroy a large variety of cancer cells each with a different genetic makeup is difficult if not impossible.

Therapies in general, then, depend upon common traits of all cancer cells (e.g., rapid cell division rate, extensive glucose uptake); or they target, especially in treatment of early stage cancers, traits that all "young" cancers' cells still retain from their originating tissue (e.g., high production of estrogen receptors in some breast cancers, high production of particular growth factor receptors in a variety of different cancers, etc.). As noted above, with time (and selection pressure coming from application of therapies) tumor cells can become resistant to particular therapies, making it even more difficult to cure the tumor. It is clear that within a tumor we can observe evidence of competition, parasitism, predation, and mutualism between clones that are coexisting and coevolving in the same tumor.

To better understand the process of cancer progression, some scientists have developed so called "oncogenetic trees" as schematic representations of the relationships that exist genetically among different tumors. These schematic trees trace the relatedness of different tumors in hopes of identifying therapies that might be useful for specific cancer "branches." For example, if a therapy works against a breast tumor with particular genetic changes, perhaps it will also destroy brain tumors that have accumulated a similar set of genetic mutations. This idea came from the phylogenetic trees that are used to tell us about the evolutionary relationships among different species, but in this case similar techniques are used to tell us about the genetic relationship of different tumors.

Cancer and Genetic Drift

Genetic drift is the frequency of a particular genetic variant in a population due to random distribution or random sampling. The process of genetic drift can best be explained by using the example of one hundred jellybeans in a jar, half of which are white and half are black, each representing a different oncogenic change in a tumor population. Randomly select a jellybean from the jar, and deposit a bean with the same color as the original that was selected into a new jar, but do not remove the selected bean from the original jar. Repeat this until there are one hundred jellybeans in the new jar. The first jar still contains the fifty-fifty mix of black and white jellybeans, but the new jar contains a random mixture of colors. If this continues multiple times (as the tumor divides continually) there will be a fluctuation in the population of jellybeans with some jars containing more blacks and others containing more whites. Eventually, it is possible that some jars will contain only blacks or only whites, totally eliminating a particular gene from the population. This process, when it involves the selection of particular genes (instead of jellybeans) is known as genetic drift.[18]

The concept of genetic drift was first developed in population genetics and was used to explain why certain genes are present in a population even though there was no selection pressure for that gene. It was "carried along" with the population as opposed to natural selection that allowed for the actual selection for positive traits and against negative traits in a given environment. Many features affect genetic drift but most prominent discussion focuses on inbreeding and cross-breeding, particularly within small or isolated populations (island populations, for example). Initially, genetic drift was seen to be counter to Darwin's ideas of natural selection, but today most molecular biologists and geneticists accept genetic drift as playing an important role in evolution.

Since cancer cells in the body (in asexually reproducing somatic cells) working together as a population seem to mimic evolution that works in populations of species, it is important to ask whether genetic drift can

18. This is described well in Wikipedia where red and blue marbles in a jar are used as a similar analogy. *Wikipedia*, s. v. "Genetic Drift."

occur in cancer cells. The answer appears to be that it does; this is based in the idea that in some tumors as many as 11,000 genetic alterations can be found but only five to seven are need to initiate the cancer. What are the rest of these mutations? Some may actually permit the tumor to survive better in that particular environment, but others appear to be random mutations that just developed in the population and continued to develop.[19] Since a larger number of random mutations occur in later stage cancers than in early cancers, it could be concluded that genetic drift plays an important role in the late evolution of the cancer in the patient.

In most of these examples relating cancer evolution to population genetics, it is noted that selection occurs at multiple levels—the level of the individual cells, the organ, the tissue, and the whole person. All the same, some mutations are "neutral" and convey no growth advantage or disadvantage to the tumor; most of these develop as a result of random mutations that continue in the population via genetic drift. There are many questions that remain about the evolution of cancers in people. These include: why are certain mutations more important in the development of cancers of some organs than others? And what is the selective pressure of the environment of a particular organ system?[20]

Summary

The mutational process that drives cancer formation and promotes its uncontrolled growth is also the main driver of evolutionary biology when it occurs in germ cells (eggs and sperm) rather than somatic cells as with cancer. The development of cancer in humans appears to be a natural process that is an inevitable result of the mutability of the human genome, which is particularly increased under certain conditions. If all DNA repair processes were perfect, evolution would not be possible—although cancer would also not be possible. Cancer is the inevitable result of the necessity of evolution for the existence of human species, with processes such as natural selection, genetic drift, and competition among clones that operate in a population's evolution likewise operating in the population of cells that make up the tumor.

19. This is described well in the work of Naugler, "Population Genetics." In this article, Naugler analyzed much of the work done with cancer genetics and points out that genetic drift and clonal evolution occur in cancer cell populations in patients.

20. For a more detailed description, see the review article by Merlo et al., "Cancer as an Evolutionary and Ecological Process."

Section 2

Chance, Necessity, Love: An Evolutionary Theology of Cancer

Chapter 4

_____

"No Exclusion of Suffering": Acceptance in a World with Cancers

Review of Section 1 and Introduction to Section 2

I n the first section, we considered the ways in which cancer is an evolutionary phenomenon of all biological being. It therefore has been present throughout all of human history. We analyzed three distinct but related dimensions of cancer: cancer as a disease of cells, as a disease of genes, and as a disease of evolutionary hallmarks. In our descriptions of how cancer cells arise from normal cells, we noted that these cells are quite precisely the "very fiber of our being," which, ironically, seek to destroy that same fiber.[1] Next, in considering cancer as a disease of genetics, we observed how the dynamisms of chance and necessity are at work in all of its molecular intricacies. And in detailing the hallmarks of cancer development, we noted how various evolutionary forces all along drive that development.

As we now consider in this second section the theological meaning of cancer as an evolutionary process, it is helpful to recognize a distinction

_____

1. From chapter 1: "In the centuries following his canonization, some Roman Catholics and some of other faiths suffering with cancers have implored Saint Peregrine to intercede on their behalf to cure them of their disease. The following is a prayer to this saint that has been employed: 'O great St. Peregrine . . . for so many years you bore in your own flesh this cancerous disease that destroys the *very fiber of our being*'" (emphasis added).

made by the existentialist philosopher, Gabriel Marcel, between what he called "problems" and "mysteries" of human being. That distinction may be summarized accordingly:

> A problem turns out to be a question, a riddle external to oneself: it is something I can put in front of me, take apart, and solve if I have the proper equipment, mental ability, perseverance, etc. A mystery is a problem in which I am involved, and in respect to which I cannot take an outsider's point of view.[2]

Up to this point, it is fair to say that we have primarily construed cancer as a "problem." That is, we have focused on it as a disease whose processes we may put in front of ourselves and then analyze (i.e., take apart and consider in detail) through scientific research. Such research certainly requires mental ability, perseverance and (much) equipment—all for the purpose of solving many cancer riddles. Approaching cancer as a problem to be solved both aims at and often achieves some very good things. Doing so allows cancer researchers to better understand the nature of the disease and cancer clinicians to employ that research to care for those suffering from it.

However, cancer may also be considered a mystery of human being for the very different but also very good purpose of our seeking out faithful understandings and wise responses to the disease. Accordingly, we may review those dimensions of cancer that we have approached as problems in order to look for mysteries within them. For example, having analyzed cancer as a cellular process in which cells turn against cells, we may pause and then ponder the fact that all cellular life—which is to say, that constituent of all of life—carries within itself the elements for its own undoing. Having described the dynamisms of chance and necessity at work in the genetics of cancers, we may reflect that chance and necessity are forces with which we must cope always and everywhere in the world. And having laid out the hallmarks of cancerous development that can threaten life, we may marvel that the same evolutionary processes directing that development may, in other circumstances, help secure new life.

Faced with such mysteries, we are led to ask this question: if God has created a world wherein the evolution of life makes possible the evolution of cancers, how may we understand the goodness of God? These questions arise: are cancers as evolutionary phenomena something that we, in faith, are called on to accept? Are they something that we, in faith, may hope will

2. Eldridge, "*Anhedonia* and the Broken World."

not always be with us? And finally: where is God and what is love given the chance and necessity at work in all dimensions of cancer?

In the chapters that follow, we shall grapple with these mysteries and others. In doing so, we will consider a variety of evolutionary theologies in order to offer responses to them. In this chapter, we will examine a theology of cancer that portrays our world as "free *to* suffer." That is, we will put forward a faith perspective along the lines of that articulated by the theologian John Polkinghorne: "the bitter presence of cancer in the world is not a sign of divine callousness or incompetence. It is the inescapable cost of a creation allowed to make itself."[3]

In chapter 5, we will consider an evolutionary theology of cancer that envisions our world as one that may be "freed *from* suffering," including that brought on by cancer. That is, we will examine a theology congruent with the following assertion of the theologian Ted Peters: "God has promised that death is going to be replaced by resurrection, and suffering will be no more."[4]

In laying out these two faithful understandings, we shall suggest that that there are, correspondingly, two types of wise responses to cancer. The response of "acceptance" or "letting-be" characterizes one type, and represents a theological appraisal of cancer as something that, as integral to life in this world, sometimes cannot be changed. The other type is distinguished by "hope" that reflects an assessment of cancer as something that both sometimes does change and even can be changed for the better of those with the disease.

In chapter 6, we will consider ways to reconcile these differing yet highly faithful perspectives and, in doing so, explain and defend the thesis of this book. We will contend that acceptance and hope are both appropriate responses to the chance and necessity of cancers, and discern how the love of God may be understood to be at work in, with, and under these evolutionary dynamisms.

The Mystery of Cancer: "No Exclusion of Chaos and Suffering"

In this world, all life processes are bound up with change and loss because all are brought into being by evolutionary chance and necessity. Given that

3. Polkinghorne, "Science and Theology," 946.
4. Peters and Hewlett, *Evolution from Creation to New Creation*, 158.

this is the way the world is, one faithful perspective on evolution calls on the faithful to have faith—that is, to trust in God and thereby accept that, given such a world, there must be various forms of natural suffering, including those brought about by a variety of cancers. That is the perspective—and the theologies that offer insights into it—that we shall consider in this chapter.

First, we will examine the work of Edward Farley as exemplary of this perspective and review some basic cancer science from our previous work, which supports this view. Next, we will intensify the implications of these cancer findings by noting that (1) because of chance, there is a statistical inevitability or necessity to there being cancers in the world, and by noting that (2) because of chance, certain cancers in individual persons may display a juggernaut quality, a near necessity, in their occurrence and in their march toward full malignancy. Given these realities, we will turn to some additional theological perspectives to look for faithful understandings of them. In doing so, we will discern a wise response in the gift to accept that, sometimes and in certain ways, cancers are things that we cannot change or may not be mutable.

To illustrate what such understandings and responses may look like, we first will look at the story of a pastor whose "letting-be" in the midst of his cancer helped him cope with that disease. Next, we will consider an account by a theologian whose understanding that the processes of life are linked to the development of this disease helped him accept the end of life that cancer brought to his spouse. We will conclude with some summary thoughts on the response of acceptance as being a faithful and wise one given the statistical inevitability of cancer's presence in this world.

"No Magic Land"

A number of theologians have reflected on how we may talk about God as good given the inescapable presence of suffering in an evolutionary world. A very small number of them have reflected on the place of cancer in such a world. Here we examine Farley's understanding of a God whose "efficacious suffering"[5] or pathos for an evolving world with its consequent cancers may bring us faith in that God and, thereby, empower us to accept, not reject this world with cancers in it. Throughout his career as a constructive theologian, the late Edward Farley distinguished himself by examining the

5. Farley, *Divine Empathy*, xvi.

mystery of human being in light of God. The following is exemplary of Farley's assessment of human existence in a world created by a good God: "Goodness of being does not exclude chaos, suffering, and tragic incompatibilities. . . . Without chaos and randomness and therefore incompatibilities and suffering, there can be no self-initiating beings, nothing available for use, and nothing that can give pleasure and meaning."[6]

Here as elsewhere, Farley abstracts the central and organizing principles at work in various realities such as congregational life, sexism, and nation/state controversies, in order to offer an ordered and coherent understanding of them. Among these realities, Farley includes cancer. "One may claim 'If there were a God, God would be able to make a world where cells do not divide and mutations do not clone themselves on the way to tumors.' Such a question can reflect disillusionment and a turn away from faith."[7] That is, Farley believes that such an assertion suggests not so much trust in God's goodness but dismay with God, given a world wherein cells may morph into malignancies.

How does Farley describe this world, both physical and biological, that we inhabit? Despite both its orderliness and obdurate facticity, the inorganic world does not bring absolute protection or security. "At work in the apparent regularities of the stars and in seemingly stable and solid 'matter' are elements of chaos." These cosmological paradoxes are heightened in the biological realm. "When life emerges, chaos (randomness, disorder) takes new and intense forms."[8] In life, randomness and disorder are the prime movers in the process of the evolution which "is the very condition of life as we know it."[9]

In producing new life forms, evolutionary processes bring about the elimination of many others, and, in this sense, all life has an inevitably tragic quality to it. By using the term *tragic*, Farley intends its precise meaning of something good that carries within itself a flaw of some sort. Thus, while we may wish that our biological world was one where life were not linked to death, in fact, "only in magic land do we find such environments."[10] That all new creations carry within themselves seeds for new suffering is exemplified in the coming to be of cancers. "Environmental contributions

6. Farley, *Good and Evil*, 149
7. Farley, "Some Preliminary Thoughts," 4.
8. Ibid., 203.
9. Farley, *Divine Empathy*, 197.
10. Ibid., 223.

aside, cancer seems to be the price we pay for being the kind of organism we are."[11] That is, our world with cancers is no magic land.

In all areas of our lives, sin shows itself not only in our clinging to things of the earth as if they could protect us from this chaos but also in our desperately demanding that the world magically conform to our desires for safety: "Guided by the conviction that because tragic finitude as contingent can be defeated, we move to defeat it. . . . Driven by this insistence, we thus move throughout times and places alert to anything that might fill our existentially hungry maws."[12] In other words, we find substitutes for God among the goods of creation—often quite superior goods such as our abilities, our well-being, the well-being of those we love—and turn them into always inadequate mini-Gods in the hope that they will secure us.

With the disease of cancer in mind, Farley writes: "In an older theology, the claim was that suffering and with it mortality was the product of the Fall, that is, sin. It may be closer to the truth to reverse it. . . . Here sin is the refusal to live in an insecure world; an inability to abide such a world; a determination to flee it into something that will secure."[13]

And who is the God who is confessed as the creator of such a world? It is the God who is the receptacle of this suffering or pathos of creation.[14] That is to say, God, the source of all beings and at work in all being, is the God of "empathy"—in the precise sense of that word in that God "senses the world's suffering." As the caring matrix of all being, this God of empathy is always at work to foster cooperation among all living things and with the world itself. "Empathy is ever an operation of enlargement, a universalization."[15] Such sensing of the suffering of the world is a primary effect of the incarnation of Christ.

In sum, Farley calls on us to accept that, given the structures of existence, there can be "no exclusion of chaos" and no world as we know it without cancers. Farley's doing so invites us to explore further what it means to live in a world that must include suffering, and as part of that suffering, must have cancers as part of its biological being. One way to begin to do so is by reviewing a variety of ways that cancers have been considered as being both an expression and aberration of normal biological being.

11. Farley, "Some Preliminary Thoughts," 1.

12. Farley, Good and Evil, 133.

13. Farley, "Some Preliminary Thoughts," 3.

14. Farley, Divine Empathy, 305.

15. Ibid., 296.

A World That Must Suffer and, therefore, Cancer

Many pithy phrases have been used to describe the disease of cancer. How-ard Varmus (who, along with J. Michael Bishop, received the Nobel prize for his research on oncogenes, and was the Director of the National Cancer Institute) has employed one: "a distorted version of our normal selves."[16] This suggests that cancer stands in contrast to normal life like a malicious Mr. Hyde to a well-meaning Dr. Jekyll, or like a monstrous Grendel to the rest of humanity.

These depictions certainly resemble those we noted earlier by Mukherjee, who construed cancer as a dangerous double or inventive copy of ourselves.[17] All of them portray cancer as a departure from what is expected and normal, and, thereby, do capture something very accurate about it. Simply put, cancer is cellular life gone awry. Here, then, is also the accuracy of considering cancer to be the quintessential disease of cells in its capacity to direct that fundamental unit of life toward what is abnormal and unexpected. Might these conceptions of cancers as distortions or as something skewed lead one to adjudge the disease to be a perversion of what is normal in life?

Farley does not view cancer this way—as a departure from the way the world both is and is meant to be—but another theologian, the Dutch-Angli-can physicist, Sjoerd Bonting, does. Bonting turns to Scripture, specifically to its headwaters in the opening verse of the book of Genesis, to argue that the watery chaos described therein not only persists alongside God's act of creation but, even afterwards, continues to disturb God's world. Bonting believes that the forces of chaos that still plague creation show themselves in particular ways, as "the physical evil of natural disasters and illness. Evil is not created, but is inherent in the remaining element of chaos."[18]

For Bonting, the disease of cancer is exemplary of this enduring cha-otic influx upon the goodness of creation. He notes that cancer is caused by "the random mutation of a single gene in one body cell, which we can consider to be a chaos event."[19] He elaborates on its processes as:

> the derailment of a very complex, orderly, coordinated function-
> ing of many genes, enzymes, hormones, messenger proteins and

16. Mukherjee, *The Emperor of All Maladies*, 363.

17. Ibid., 388.

18. Bonting, *Chaos Theology*, 23.

19. Ibid.

receptors existing in our body cells under normal conditions. This order has been established by the Creator in the course of evolutionary creation and is established anew in each individual, owing to the genetic system present in its cells. A chaos event, the random mutation of one gene in one cell, can make this order degenerate to chaos on the cellular level.[20]

There is a truth more than poetic in this portrayal of cancer as a disease caused by chaos. Certainly it is accurate to claim that cancers co-opt many of the normal processes of cellular life, as we saw earlier in the ways cancerous cells employ the Warburg Effect to direct energy away from normal growth and towards their abnormal proliferation. Rather than engaging in a wholesale invention of novel strategies, cancer cells adapt and reshape the strategies that maintain normalcy by twisting these processes to the singular, asocial purpose of their own survival and proliferation/increase.

And yet, it is closer to the precise truth to say that chaos is not so much the first cause as it is an end result of cancers, for there is nothing aberrant about the forces or mechanisms out of which they arise. That is, this "derailment of cellular order," even with its often awful consequences, derives from and progresses according to nothing other than normal cellular ways of being. Cancer is a natural and inevitable outcome of the way that we are made up of cells, and the way in which all individual cells are made: vulnerable and not quite perfect. Indeed, as we have noted earlier, that which is co-opted or hijacked in the process of oncogenesis by the Rous sarcoma virus is something locatable within the normal cell itself. Cancers come into being by alterations to our own genes, our own selves (sometimes carried to us by viruses).

The fault of our cancers lies not outside us, but within our inherent genetic endowment that, ironically, brings about all of the good that we are. Our cells, the basis of life, have within themselves the elements of their own undoing of life in the form of genes that control what cells are and what they are destined to become. As these elements assemble by chance, they are carried along by the same law-like regularities that govern all rapidly growing normal forms of cellular life—including, as we noted earlier, wound healing and the growth of microorganisms. And as they assemble into tumors in our bodies and seek out the sustenance of blood, they behave like bodily organs—except that, unlike organs, cancerous tumors enlist support for their own sake, not for the common good of our bodies.

20. Ibid.

The "chaos" of cancer, then, is less the source and more the outcome of the driving process of all life: evolution through natural selection. Since it comes about through natural selection, certain classical terms of Darwinian evolution therefore do apply to its development: cancer is the product of a single clone that beats out the odds against its survival. It is the mass of cells that have excelled at doing what life does best—thriving amidst adversity. Cancer, then, is not alien to life, but exemplifies life's Darwinian features. The disease arises when that which evolutionary forces produce— growth, change, and novelty—occur at the expense of that which evolution also often brings about—stasis, regularity, and harmony.

Accordingly, the term *tragic* that Farley uses to describe all of life is very appropriate to apply to the development of cancers—in the sense that cancerous development is a flaw at the base of life or a defect hardwired into its cellular base of being that may cause it to fail. Here is another way to say this: within the drive of life for new life may be found that which may cut short lives. Therefore, just as it is not hyperbole to claim that cancer is the quintessential disease of cells, likewise it may be accurately assessed as the quintessential disease of life, in the sense that it is the disorder that comes about through the very processes by which all life comes about.

Because of Chance, the Necessity of Cancer

While cancers are not alien to, but a part of, life, does that mean that they are *necessarily* a part of life—that is, because of life, there must be cancers? The answer might seem to be "no," for this reason: if all individual cancers come about through chance mutations—that is, through changes in DNA structure that may occur but do not have to do so—then it might seem that there is no necessity that any will come about.

However, while there is no absolute necessity for the existence of cancers, there appears to be a statistical inevitability to their occurring somewhere, sometime. There are a variety of ways in which this truth might be explicated, but a very familiar example—coin tossing—clearly illustrates why this is so. Each time a coin is tossed, the odds are fifty percent that it will come up "tails." However, the more times it is flipped, the odds increase that one of those times it will turn up "tails." This happens because, in all games of chance, there is also at work a law-like regularity—the law of large numbers. Those running gambling establishments against whom money is waged know that while their "house of games" may lose heavily in one or several placed bets, it is predictable that their enterprise will succeed as the games go on. Hence the adage that, in the long run, "the house always wins."

Within a cell, there are more nuanced and refined conditions than those directing the inanimate world of flipped coins that govern life and, thereby, strengthen the inevitability of cancerous happenstances. To be sure, the odds that a single mutation of DNA will initiate a malignant process within a cell are very small. But trillions of mutations are occurring worldwide as we write this sentence and as you read it. Accordingly, it is a statistical certainty that a malignancy will develop somewhere, sometime—and is doing so as you read this sentence. Indeed, this inexorable quality to cancer becomes apparent when one looks at the mutational load over the course of an individual lifespan in the vast numbers of dividing cells that are undergoing these mutations. So while cancer is an extremely rare disease, it happens as the cumulative consequence of the 10,000 trillion cells divisions that occur in the average lifetime.

Accordingly, it is also statistically inevitable that on average each human being will experience at least one cancer per lifetime. For example, in one particular site of origin—the prostate—we know that 80 percent of males over age eighty develop cancers there. This statistical loading of life for cancerous outcomes is why Greaves employs gaming metaphors about cancer and evolution.

Greaves is not alone in using evocative images to describe the persistence of cancer. In his 2011 article, "On the Intrinsic Inevitability of Cancer: From Foetal to Fatal Attraction," Sui Huang writes, "in summary, at least cancer initiation, the cell intrinsic process of malignant transformation, seems to be inevitable—a fact that will motivate our discourse on the profound link between development and tumorigenesis and on the stochastic nature of the initiating events."[21] Huang's point is one that summarizes ours: within the flow of life itself, there is a pull like gravity toward the development of cancers.

Because of Chance, the Necessity of Some Individual Cancers

Earlier, we noted that not all cells that start out on the road to cancerous progression succeed at becoming true or full cancers. So far as cancerous

21. Huang, "On the Intrinsic Inevitability of Cancer," 816.

cells are concerned, that road is full of many obstacles that may and often do block their way forward. Also, some cancers that do succeed in becoming true cancers may not cause much danger. And other cancers may, effectively, cease to be—sometimes spontaneously and, in an increasing number of instances, through medical interventions. Consequently, cancer incidence and cancer mortality are separable phenomena—which is to say that having cancer does not necessarily mean that one will die from it.

And yet, cancer incidence and cancer mortality are clearly related phenomena: for some people with the disease—in fact, slightly under half of all those diagnosed with one of its many forms—do eventually die from it. And a select portion of these cancers also display what may be described as a juggernaut quality—an inexorable and unstoppable feature to their development. These cells do so because, by chance, they have gained special advantages that alter their genetic programming and enable them to cobble together unique ways of circumventing normal rules for communal and cooperative cellular life.

It is a hallmark feature of cancer cells that as they progress toward a malignant state they become increasingly genetically unstable and that the downstream consequence of their doing so is that they will evolve more rapidly. It is the evolutionary underpinnings of cancers that account for such this progression. That is, through natural selection certain cancers might progress to a better-adapted state in which they can take fuller advantage of the hosts in which they are growing. Like a quickening spiral, genetic instability breeds further instability—new mutations accumulate faster—leading more quickly and more assuredly to new adaptations. This accelerated evolution thus produces a richer "keyboard" upon which natural selection can play to produce those cancers that are most successful and, therefore, most difficult to treat. The outcome of evolutionary forces that achieve malignancy is very often a state of biological robustness, which means that the cancer has reached a hardiness by which it co-opts the body's mechanisms for its own sake and, likewise for its own good, can defend itself from host defenses.[22] In such circumstances, new challenges to the cancer in the form of chemotherapy and radiation may kill the vast majority of cancer cells, but it is the norm that relapses for such cancers do occur and that "cure is still rare."[23]

22. Kitano, "Cancer as a Robust System."
23. Ibid., 227.

Thus, relapse is a common outcome of many treatment modalities. As we have noted, rare cancer stem cells exhibit enhanced robustness, allowing them to linger and lurk unaffected by standard therapies only to burst forth after a period of quiescence.[24] For unknown reasons, cancer stem cells are often more resistant to chemotherapy and radiation.[25] Moreover, many older chemotherapies, and even some newer anti-cancer drugs represent agents of natural selection that, while eliminating most cancer cells, will create a bottleneck or a filter through which rare resistant cells will pass and, ultimately, end the life of the host.

In the previous section, we concluded that the appearance of cancers in this world appears to be inevitable. In this section, we have noted that the progress of certain individual cancers may be close to inevitable. In these senses, we may say that cancer is something that is not mutable or cannot be changed.

Cancer as Something that Cannot be Changed: Some Practical Theological Considerations

Among the questions we posed early on in the introduction of this practical theological inquiry of cancer was this one: is cancer something that can be changed? We may now attempt to provide an answer. If by this question we are asking whether the fact may be changed that there always have been, are now, and, in this world, always will be cancers, then the answer appears to be "no." While not all cancers that occur must do so, it seems that, sooner or later, there must be some occurrences. Similarly, if by this question we are asking whether the developmental track of certain "juggernaut" cancers that have been initiated may be substantially altered, it seems that the answer likewise is "no." Some people with cancer do report that they have inklings of this unchangeable aspect of the disease in experiencing their own as having something like of a life of its own—which, in a real sense, all cancers do.

As a practical theological inquiry, we are led to ask: what is a faithful understanding of God given that the disease of cancer is, in the senses described above, something that cannot be changed? During his career, Farley offered an understanding intended to produce faith in the goodness of God amidst the suffering produced by an evolutionary world of chance

24. Clevers, "The Cancer Stem Cell."
25. Hanahan and Weinberg, "Hallmarks" (2011), 646.

and change that may be summarized this way: the world that God created has suffering built into it.

A cluster of theologians have offered similar theological positions. Reflecting on the fact that life requires the mutation of germ lines in order to produced new species, John Polkinghorne remarks:

> It is inevitable also that somatic cells, body cells, will also be able to mutate genetically, and sometimes when they do they will become malignant: you can't have the one without the other. And that, I think, is a mildly helpful insight for us. Of course the existence of cancer is a deeply anguishing fact about the world and I don't wish for a minute to diminish the feeling of anguish or indeed anger that we feel at that fact, but at least the scientific insight of evolution shows us that it is not gratuitous. It is not something that if God was a bit more careful, or a bit less callous, could easily have eliminated. It is the inescapable shadow side of a world in which creatures make themselves.[26]

How may God be pronounced as good while permitting such suffering? Polkinghorne has several strategies for addressing this question, but derives a central one from Paul's Letter to the Philippians about Christ:

> who, though he was in the form of God, did not regard equality with God as something to be exploited, but emptied himself, taking the form of a slave, being born in human likeness. And being found in human form, he humbled himself and became obedient to the point of death—even death on a cross (NRSV 2:6-8).

The key phrase in this passage regarding Christ is that he "emptied himself," from the Greek *kenosen* for "to empty." And the key feature about these verses of Scripture for our evolutionary theology of cancer is that they derive not from a tragic chorus, but, before they were included in Scripture, may very well have been verses of a joyful hymn in the church.[27]

Along with Polkinghorne, theologian and scientist George Murphy discerns in these verses a song of praise to the God who, through Christ, does not hold on to power over particular occurrences in the world: "kenosis means that God does not cling to privileges of divinity and insist upon credit for creative work."[28] To be sure, Murphy notes that there are many complexities in this creation. "We are baffled by the extinctions of splendid

26. Polkinghorne, "Does God Interact?"

27. Martin, *A Hymn of Christ*; Yarbro Collins, "Psalms, Philippians 2:6-11."

28. Murphy, *The Cosmos*, 104.

creatures, the growth of cancer in someone we love, or ethical choices that seem to have no right answer."[29] But he employs this chorale of God's taking on the lowly form of a servant in order to account for such complexities. "Kenosis does not mean God's abdication but God working in a way that is not recognizable to theologians of glory."[30]

Here, Murphy invokes the language of his Lutheran tradition, wherein "theologies of glory" refer, among other things, to sometimes well-meaning but always mistaken efforts to pinpoint God's actions in the world. In this schema, theologies of the cross—that is, theologies like that invoked by language of God's kenosis—propose that God's oversight of the world cannot be clearly discerned by the eye or demonstrated through reason. "In some cases we can explain why a natural disaster has happened or why one person rather than another develops cancer, but this is not always the case."[31]

Murphy favors an understanding of God's creating kenotically not only for the consoling understandings it provides regarding the way the cosmos works, but for the favor God thereby bestows on the cosmos itself. Thus, Murphy proposes that God was certainly present during the enigmatic early minutes of creation, but adds. "God's kenosis means that we do not expect to observe astronomical phenomena that science *cannot* explain," because "kenosis means that God does not cling to privileges of divinity and insist upon credit for creative work."[32]

Murphy considers a classic musical work in order to illustrate the blessing God bestows on God's handiwork. "Perhaps Haydn captured the right note in *The Creation*. In it God's initial command for the creation of light is almost a whisper, 'And God spoke: Let there be light! And there was'—and then comes a powerful 'LIGHT' and a joyous blaze of music. The thunder of creation drowns out the still, small voice of the creator."[33] Just as in Haydn's oratorio the soft voice of the creator gives way to the powerful voice of created light, so God gives way to both creation and the sciences that strive to apprehend it. In so doing, Murphy avers, God gracefully gives glory to both.

Given these faithful understandings of creation and cancer, what might be a wise response—that is, what might be a way of being in the world that

29. Ibid., 5.
30. Ibid., 81.
31. Ibid., 87.
32. Ibid., 102, 104.
33. Ibid., 105.

might enable us to live in it prudently and well? If it is a fact that cancer is, in the senses we have explored, something that cannot be changed, and if it is also true that the whys and wherefores of this disease may not always be clear, then, in keeping with the wisdom of the well-known Serenity Prayer, we suggest that some kind of "acceptance" be a part of that response.

Of course, in singling out "acceptance," we have in mind a response informed by the Serenity Prayer not only to cancers but to all other things over which we do not have control. To illustrate what such a response might look in religious life, we first will share the story of a retired pastor who reflected on the meaning of *Gelassenheit*, or acceptance in the form of "letting-be," to explain how he tried to make religious sense of his experience with his own cancer. Next, we will share the story of a theologian who, in coming to accept the evolutionary nature of cancer came to accept the death that cancer brought to someone he loved.

A Case Study of *Gelassenheit*:
The Theology of the Cross and Cancer

At the time he told the story of how he coped with cancer, Charles was a sixty-nine-year-old married man with one adult child, and a retired pastor of the Evangelical Lutheran Church in America. He shared that "after a lifetime of good health," he experienced several illnesses including a life-threatening diagnosis of prostate cancer: "There's something kind of ludicrous about the whole thing when one looks at it. Well, first of all, what they do to you. What it means to be cut up and slashed open. I got scars from my chin to my pubic bone. And what a ridiculous thing to go through when you think about it—that they make you well by tearing you up."[34]

Yet, in the midst of his suffering, Charles found comfort in his faith that helped him accept and cope with his cancer. "Faith tells you that it's all right what you're experiencing. It is all right. It is all right. And, that doesn't mean it's pleasant. And, there is no relief where you say, And, see, consolation was there before you began."[35]

In thinking back on his long and productive life, and then on the surprise of a life-threatening illness at his retirement, Charles found a resource for comfort in a set of hymns. "What they all had is what the Mennonites

34. In Hummel, *Clothed in Nothingness*, 56.
35. Ibid., 57.

call *Gelassenheit*. This means, not a resignation. It's a kind of a way of saying, letting go, letting God. . . . No, no, it's not Stoicism."[36]

What does Charles mean by this term, *Gelassenheit*? It is usually translated much the way Charles interprets it: as the state of mind/heart of "letting be" or "letting go" in the face of adversity. And whether it was Christof Friedrich Oetinger (1702–1782) or Reinhold Niebuhr (1892–1971), who composed the now world-famous Serenity Prayer, in its German version *Gelassenheit* is the equivalent for the English word "acceptance." Charles rightly notes its central place within the Mennonite tradition as a "yielding" to sufferings in the world. Furthermore, he is quite accurate in identifying the central importance of *Gelassenheit* for Mennonites where its literal meaning of "letting go" or "letting be" has often encouraged members of its churches to endure threats without and stresses within.

A reflective pastor, Charles offered the following elaborations on what his own experience of *Gelassenheit* related to accepting his prostate cancer:

> And I would say that *Gelassenheit* almost sounds like Stoicism. And I think Stoicism falls short because Stoicism seems like metaphysical sour grapes where people say, "Well, these things aren't all that hot, and life itself isn't all that hot, so what can I expect?" But, *Gelassenheit* means, ". . . I'm just going to give myself over to a larger reality. I don't pretend to understand and I don't want to understand. I don't have to understand. There's no fight and things are all right."[37]

Charles reports that he has had no recurrences of his cancer. Following his recovery, he also shared that he became involved in a prostate support group and explained his reason for doing so this way: "I appreciate the good I got from modern medicine. . . . I owe, I owe."[38]

In her work, *God and the Web of Creation*, Ruth Page employs the concept of *Gelassenheit* much the way that Polkinghorne, Murphy, and others have employed kenosis—as a way of signifying God's power in this world by God's empowering and permitting the world to be something other than God. "'Letting be' is a suggestive phrase for God allowing to come into being a world which has its own character. . . . It retains the performative ring of the Hebrew 'yehi or', that is 'Let there be light.'"[39] Following Page's

36. Ibid., 82.
37. Ibid.
38. Ibid.,112.
39. Page, *God and the Web of Creation*, 5.

schema, one does not look to God for answers to the whys and wherefores of diseases like cancer, but looks for ways, as Charles has done, to care for others who suffer from it.

How may we make religious sense of the way Charles accepts his disease? Of course, there are many ways we might do so, but one would be to reflect on how *he* does so: from his understanding of a kenotic "theology of the cross." As he reflected on his experience with cancer and his experiences of God during that experience, Charles claimed he can never clearly discern God's revelation in the world throughout all this because "God is found in the cross." For Charles, the theology of the cross did not explain to him how God was at work in his cancer. "To look for God means you are not going to find him because God—this is what I think—God is found on the cross." It does appear that "letting go" of efforts to discern God's will in the world enabled Charles to accept that God was with him in ways that transcended his understanding and helped him focus on being with others: "I didn't focus on God's actions when I was sick."[40]

A Case Study of Acceptance: Dancing with the Sacred at the End of Life

At the beginning of his book, *Dancing with the Sacred: Evolution, Ecology, and God*, theologian Karl Peters states his intent to look throughout his work "for a more integrated understanding of God and evolutionary theory, of God working creatively in the world and of Darwin's theory of random variation and natural selection."[41] Having surveyed various evolutionary phenomena in the world around us, he makes a specific reference toward the end of his book to cancer. What he "came to realize was that cancer cells are an example of Darwinian evolution. The cells of our body mutate all the time. . . . Random variations and natural selection occur not just in the transmission of genes from one generation to the next. They occur within the confines of our own bodies."[42]

The impetus for Peters's appreciation of the evolutionary nature of cancer was an event in his own life: the diagnosis of his wife, Carol, with a rare stomach cancer that had metastasized and, eventually, led to her death. "What meaning can we find in a world of chance and necessity?" Peters

40. In Hummel, *Clothed in Nothingness*, 96.
41. Peters, *Dancing with the Sacred*, 1.
42. Ibid., 114.

asks at the end of his book as he tries to construct a theological understanding of cancers and of the cancer that brought about the death of his wife.[43]

Peters's approach to all evolutionary phenomena exemplifies a "naturalist theology" with a "non-personal" understanding of God: "as a naturalistic theist I do not deny that God is more than the world, but I do want to focus continually on how we can know and be related to God in our natural world."[44] Working out this particular understanding of the relationship between God and the world, Peters claims, "while I think of God as a sacred dance that continuously gives rise to new possibilities for existence and selects some of those to continue, I realize that loss and suffering are also a result of this process."[45] Throughout his work, therefore, Peters articulates his faith in a God who, in allowing for many possibilities in the unfolding of life, also has permitted Darwinian developments like cancers to be inevitable. Indeed, he claims that "to err is divine" because "biological creation takes place by making mistakes."[46] Cancer is one of those creations:

> Some genetic changes lead to new forms of life. However, the vast majority of biological maturations lead to malfunctioning organisms, sterility, and death. The results of cell changes in our bodies that cause runaway cell growth can create suffering and death. But the system of evolution that embodies constant change also has created our living planet, our species, ourselves. . . . Theologically, this means for me that I cannot regard cancer as evil, even though it caused suffering and death for me and someone I love.[47]

Like the disciples of Jesus immediately following the crucifixion, Peters contends that we live in a world where the fact and power of the resurrection are not always discernible. At the same time, Peters contemplates the death of Jesus not only in order to ponder how death is connected to life, but in order to hope for something beyond death. "The universe seems to be so constituted that one cannot separate creation from destruction, pleasure from pain, joy from sorrow. . . . In the center of sorrow there can be profound joy. Even during the dying of a loved one, new love can be born."[48]

43. Ibid., 131.
44. Ibid., vii.
45. Ibid., viii.
46. Ibid., 40.
47. Ibid., 114.
48. Ibid., 118.

Peters claims that the birth of such love came about as Carol and he coped with her diagnosis of a cancer that could not be cured:

> Because we had no hope of life, we experienced a strange kind of freedom. It was the freedom of knowing that the worst was going to happen, so we could do whatever we wanted. . . . Most importantly, we talked. We reviewed our life together. We enjoyed remembering the good times and we came to terms with all the trouble we had caused to one another. We talked, we listened, we forgave. As life was ebbing away, love was growing.[49]

Both Carol and Karl were transformed by Carol's dying over a period of fifteen months. She, the extrovert, "learned just to be." Peters shared the following particularly poignant story of her doing so. "She learned to sit in her Lazy-boy on the porch, being by me through her feeding tube, and looking out at our yard and lake. One day she was rewarded. She saw an eagle drop out of the sky into the lake, catch a fish, and fly with it right over our house."[50]

While the plummeting of eagles on prey below may be a beautiful sight to behold, we also believe that it exemplifies the evolutionary struggle of all biological existence. Throughout his book, Peters searches out the beautiful work of God within all evolutionary phenomena. As the story above indicates, Peters was spiritually transformed as he came to understand and accept the evolution of cancer, not just in the abstract but in the very being and body of his beloved spouse. Other blessings came his way that affirmed his sense that life could come out of death, including the invitation to conduct a wedding for the daughter of two good friends after his wife's memorial service. "I felt the spirit of love, which had grown so rich during Carol's dying, was now present for me in this couple as they took their vows to become husband and wife. In that ceremony, I experienced resurrection."[51]

Conclusion

In considering a wise response to the inevitability of natural suffering, Farley employs a term that may be even more powerful than the term

49. Ibid., 117.
50. Ibid.
51. Ibid., 124.

acceptance and which we understand to witness to the goodness of God in a world with phenomena such as cancers in it. That term is *consent*. "Consent is the existential and emotional acknowledgment of the propriety of these things. Consent does not demand an elimination of resistance to suffering of all kinds or a repression of the desire of elementary passions through or past mundane goods."[52]

Living in a world whose physical and biological structures do not promise what Farley calls "security," the gospel promise comes to us, and, in hearing it, we become "founded." Here, consent also involves not only the serenity to accept that cancers are often things that do not or cannot be changed, but also means having the courage to change something within ourselves: to turn from sinful non-acceptance of the world, even with its cancers, toward an embrace of it. "Once the self is founded by the presence of the sacred, it is not turned away from the world (as in refusal) but turned toward the world as a venturing of the self amidst the perils of the world."[53]

Farley suggests what such consent might mean for all of us facing a world with cancers in it. "I would submit that when Good News is proclaimed, the human being can accept the real tragic-comic world—to enjoy its beauty and help people victimized by it. A practical theology of cancer, and the response to cancer would have as part of it its empowering release into world acceptance."[54] We are reminded in these words of Charles's account of letting go, of his thereby being opened up to the world around himself, and his consequent care for others with cancer.

We may understand the wise response of acceptance of a world with cancers in it to be connected with consent to all limits on life in this world— limits that include the reality of death. Given the inevitability of death and that in this world there can be no exclusion of chaos and suffering, one wise response would certainly be to accept the world as it is, to have empathy for it and to have empathy for inevitable suffering of all living things in it. Certainly, this response of acceptance is compelling and, we aver, is a faithful one.

But we are left wondering: does this one wise response exhaust all possible responses to a world with such limits? We think not.

---

52. Farley, *Good and Evil*, 149.

53. Ibid., 150.

54. Farley, "Some Preliminary Thoughts," 5.

To indicate why not, we first reflect on these words of the philosopher of religion Holmes Rolston III, which echo the responses we have described in this chapter:

> . . . a tragic view of life, but one in which tragedy is the shadow of prolific creativity. . . . [T]he biological sciences—evolutionary history, ecology, molecular biology—can be brought to support this view, although neither tragedy nor creativity are part of their ordinary vocabulary. Since the world we have, in its general character, is the only world logically and empirically possible under the natural givens on Earth . . . *this world that is, ought to be.*[55]

This view is very much like that put forward by Karl Peters, and we believe that there is much about it that is commendable.

But we may contrast this view with the perspective put forth by another theologian, Ted Peters: "to conflate a natural condition with an imperative—an *ought*—is fallacious."[56] While Ted Peters argues against such conflations by appealing to the many and varied various philosophical claims that just because something is a certain way does not mean that it ought to be that way, his strongest warrant for his rejection of the naturalness of suffering in the world is theological:

> The tendency among theistic evolutionists . . . to see violence, suffering, and death as merely natural and hence value-neutral—represents a failure of theological nerve. . . . *God has promised that death is going to be replaced by resurrection, and suffering will be no more.* From the theological point of view, we simply cannot let science alone define what is natural, or, worse, redefine violence, suffering, and death as value neutral.[57]

In the next chapter, we will examine another and distinctive theological take on making meaning of the mystery of human being in a world with cancers in it. This other position, like that we have described in this section is actually not a single theology but a variety of theologies. But all of them cluster in their expressing a deep dis-ease—with the presence of suffering in the natural world brought on by diseases like cancer. And though not all of them directly consider cancer, taken together they seem to advance proposals something like these: we accept that this is a world with cancers

---

55. Rolston III, "Naturalizing and Systematizing Evil," 85; emphasis added.
56. Peters and Hewlett, *Evolution from Creation to New Creation,* 175.
57. Ibid., 158; emphasis added.

in them—and that this world and the God who created it are good. But we also trust—or more accurately, hope—that God has something better in mind, or has a promise of something more, than this world with cancers in it.

We will begin our inquiry in the following chapter by looking more closely at the thought of Ted Peters—to whom (and not to Karl Peters) all references to "Peters" in the remainder of our book are intended. While he does not directly consider the disease of cancer, Peters proposes that God intends something more than this world with its suffering, loss, and death—realities that may be brought on by a disease like cancer. And, as we do so, we will be mindful of a scriptural passage that is key to Peters's thought and to our proposals for a theology of hope in a world with cancers:

> See, the home of God is among mortals. He will dwell with them as their God; they will be his peoples, and God himself will be with them; he will wipe every tear from their eyes. Death will be no more; mourning and crying and pain will be no more, for the first things have passed away (Rev 21:3b–4, NRSV).

Chapter 5

Something More: Hope in a World of Cancer Chance and Necessity

I n chapter 4, we examined a number of compelling religious perspectives that together more or less propose that God has created a world in which there are and must be cancers, and that, in accepting this, we may become empowered to be part of the redemptive work of God in bearing the sufferings brought on by cancers. We concluded that these theologies offer a manifestly faithful understanding of and concomitantly wise response to both the goodness of God and the presence of cancers in this world.

Now we will focus on a largely different theological perspective on the mystery of cancer: God has something more in mind than this world with its occurrences of cancer. We will begin by highlighting certain key ideas offered by the theologian Ted Peters on the suffering brought on by various evolutionary events in this world and on God's intent to end such suffering in a redeemed world. With these notions in mind, we will examine some perspectives that suggest, in the redeemed time to come, cancer will become a thing of the past. We will conclude that, while most of these proposals for God's cancer-free future appear upon careful analysis to be incoherent, we may nevertheless hope that God intends to deliver this world from cancers—though exactly how, we do not know.

Accordingly, we will return to the philosophy of Gabriel Marcel and introduce the theological cancer memoirs of Deanna Thompson for understandings of hope in God's goodness even if we may lack clear evidence around us for such hoping. Furthermore, we will argue that, with the eyes of faith, we may discern something of God's good intent for the future from certain current "cancer facts": (1) not all mutations that might initiate cancerous development will do so; (2) not even all those cells that do begin to develop such deadly abilities will succeed in attaining those capacities; (3) many events that might contribute to mutagenesis and thereby initiate cancers themselves may be prevented. Finally, we will indicate a resource for faithful hoping, in that sometimes hoping for change to the suffering of cancers may contribute to their changing both through the consequent development of better treatments and by the seeking out of such treatments by the hopeful.

Epigenesis: Hope for God's Creation After Genesis

In *Evolution from Creation to New Creation*, Peters asks:

> can theological affirmations of divine love and omnipotence be reconciled with what Charles Darwin called "waste," namely, the eons and eons of deep time in which animals of prey suffered at the hand of predators, in which sentient beings suffered from disease and disaster, in which 98% of all species have perished?[1]

Peters's short answer is that, while we may detect no godly intent operative in natural suffering, we can discern God's good purpose for this world in God's promise to end all suffering in a time to come. "The natural world of which we are so much a part is not the only reality. There is more. Transformation is coming. The transformation brought by the new creation will redefine the old creation; it will reorient the present history of evolution."[2]

Throughout his work, Peters elaborates on God's promise to reign in this new world by removing the natural suffering found in the current one. What kind of a new creation does Peters thereby envision? It may appear to be much like Farley's perfect and, therefore, not so good world in which "there can be no competition [and] every entity is invulnerable not only to pain but to frustration."[3] Yet, it is precisely what appears to be Farley's "magic land" without ills that Peters proposes that God promises to bring forth. "The new creation will be a physical creation, even if it is pervaded

---

1. Peters and Hewlett, *Evolution from Creation to New Creation*, 118.

2. Ibid., 27–28.

3. Farley, "Some Preliminary Thoughts," 2–3.

by the divine Spirit . . . (Rev 21:4). The violence, suffering, and death so inescapable in Darwin's world will become only a past memory."[4]

Peters believes that the present world is good, but, with its current sources of suffering, it is not yet as good as it shall be. "God creates from the future, not the past. God starts with redemption and then draws creation toward it. Or, perhaps better said, God's ongoing creative work is also God's redeeming work. Only a redeemed creation will be worthy of the appellation 'very good.'"[5] It is this "very good" creation that Peters proposes as God's purpose for a suffering creation: "The abiding divine activity of continuing to provide the world with an open future we refer to as continuing creation, *creatio continua*."[6] Whether God will remake the current world or create a new one is unclear. But, for Peters, what is certain is that God's will is for a better world.

In order to account for how God will later create over and above what God has brought forth in the genesis of this world, Peters appeals to the philosophical and theological concept of "epigenesis," which derives "from the Greek, *genesis* mean[ing] 'to create or generate,' and *epi* means 'again or on top of.' Thus, *epigenesis* refers to ongoing creativity. Rather than assume that everything is governed by the way the world began, we affirm epigenetic newness as every day's new possibility."[7] Broadly speaking, then, epigenesis refers to the openness of the world to that which is not yet in the world. It points to the fact that things in the world may emerge that we might have a very hard time predicting from or predicating upon that which has preceded them.[8] Given the development of various phenomena through epigenesis, we are led to ask: Under the guidance of God, could the nature of life itself be so transformed, whether gradually or rapidly, that it might become one without cancers? Peters does not ask this question, as he does not specifically list the elimination of sicknesses among the attributes of a newly ordered and transformed world. Indeed, like many other constructive theologians who propose good news about the end of time, Peters does not detail much of what he expects will occur at that time.

4. Peters and Hewlett, *Evolution from Creation to New Creation*, 162.

5. Ibid., 160.

6. Ibid., 161.

7. Ibid., 162.

8. Cf. Waddington, "The Epigenotype"; Moss, "From Representational Preformationism"; van Speybroeck, "From Epigenesis to Epigenetics," 79: epigenetics refers to the science of "those interactions of genes with their environment that bring the phenotype into being."

However, another theologian, Robert John Russell, does offer some specifics that suggest that cancers will be absent. "An acceptable eschatology must . . . include the curing of disease and the overcoming of death. *The reality of disease and death is shared by all multi-cellular life on earth. The scope of God's eschatological redemption must therefore be co-terminus with it.*"[9] Russell uses the term, "natural evil," as did Bonting earlier, to describe the presence of suffering in the world brought on by diseases to multi-cellular organisms.[10] However, he conceives of these disorders as evil, not because they are contrary to the order of original creation, but because they are contrary the nature of God's redeemed creation in a time to come.

But while we can hope for and even imagine such a new order of things, might we be able to provide a plausible and coherent description of this world? And what does the answer to this question mean for the hope of a world without the one disorder that arises specifically because of our multi-cellularity—the disease of cancer?

A World to Come without Cancers: Not a Magic Land but a Promised Land

Previously we concluded that given the conditions of this world—that is, given the life of cells and the inevitability of genetic mutations—this world is one in which cancers must occur. But what of a transformed world that has been not so much described as fondly hoped and fervently prayed for by Peters and others? Are there any indications in this world that a new one might come into being, and in doing so, that the bond between the development of life and the development of cancers might be broken? Or to ask this differently: are there any indications from the way this world is ordered now for how it might be reconstituted in the future?

Perhaps we might look for indications of the possible end of the evolutionary disease of cancer within the phenomenon of biological evolution itself. What if the world itself were to evolve so that its very fabric were to change? Might not the process of "continuous creation" itself give us hope that a biological world might come to pass in which cancers were not present?

Our impetus to ask these questions arises from the above theological portrayals of a world without suffering. Peters and Russell are joined in this

9. Russell, "The Groaning of Creation," 139–40; emphasis added.
10. Ibid.

envisioning by an exemplary "theologian of hope," Jürgen Moltmann, who describes a redeemed world as one in which those natural laws that bind up our aeon will be undone and who finds warrant for his hope in the indeterminacy of current sub-atomic processes: the coming kingdom of glory would not a closed system, but "an open system."[11] Because he proposes that life in the end time will not be subject to the limitations of this time, Moltmann envisions that there will be "change without transience, time without the past, and life without death."[12]

Theologians of hope like Moltmann support their proposals of a time to come freed from death not only with their readings of current science but by often referring to the new creation as portrayed in Revelation 21. Depictions of creatures not visiting their typical destruction on one another are to be found in elsewhere in Scripture:

> The wolf shall live with the lamb, the leopard shall lie down with the kid, the calf and the lion and the fatling together, and a little child shall lead them. The cow and the bear shall graze, their young shall lie down together; and the lion shall eat straw like the ox (Isa 11:6–7).

However, Christopher Southgate, a theologian who has written much about suffering in nature both in our times and in hoped-for end times, discerns problems of coherence in notions that nature might ever be exempt from it. In doing so, Southgate reflects on the first verse of the Scripture above: "it is very hard to see how the leopardness of leopards could be fulfilled in eschatological coexistence with kids."[13] Southgate's concerns arise from his conviction that all creatures have unique ways of being that are more or less constitutive of what and who they are, and, consequently, how they behave. Therefore, he finds it hard to conceive how any assembly of wolves and lambs would not ultimately constitute a community of pain and suffering.

Can we conceive of a peaceable kingdom in a redeemed time to come among cellular communities in which none of its cells are destroying other ones in a cancerous manner? In a sense, the answer is yes, for we can conceive that, in a time to come, genes might still very much be genes and not undergo mutations within individual cells that will bring about the death of others. We can conceive of genes not mutating and initiating cancers

---

11. Moltmann, *Science and Wisdom*, 47.

12. Ibid., 46.

13. Southgate, "Creation as 'Very Good,'" 83.

then because it happens all the time now. As we have noted throughout our inquiry, such cellular harmony is, in fact, the norm of biological being.

Nevertheless, it is hard to conceive of life, whether in this world or in any one to come, without energy, motion, and concomitant contact; and it is precisely such physical activities that inevitably alter the structure of genes and thereby initiate oncogenesis. The inevitability of cancerous occurrences, not only in this life but in any kind of existence, is not, to paraphrase Southgate, due to the cellularity of cells or genetics of genes—that is, in the ways cells are constituted and that genes work. Rather, the necessity for cancers lies in the physical forces that operate on genes and cells. Consequently, it is hard not only to conceive of but even to picture life—if we would wish to still call it life—in a time to come that would not have cancers.

That natural forces, even those operative in a redeemed nature, would inevitably contribute to occurrences of some kind of cancerous processes seems to be entailed in the reflections of another theologian, Wesley Wildman, on Isaiah 11:7. "Thus, even if Isaiah's vision of the lion eating straw like the ox were to come true, we would still have suffering in nature, especially in the form of plant injury and accidents."[14] Here we hear themes similar to those proposed by Farley—that suffering and disturbances are built into the structure of existence. Even carefully constructed philosophical proposals that, in a redeemed world, creatures might no longer obtain their sustenance through the death of other creatures but, rather, be resourced by the emanation of light do not remove this problem, for the occurrence of such light, "would still leave accident and injury and possibly disease to worry about."[15] We do not know what kind of light-induced diseases Wildman has in mind, but cancerous melanomas come to our minds—for light produces energy and it is perturbations produced by energy that bring about much natural suffering, and, typically, is the first cause in this particular kind of cancer.

To be sure, one might hope that, in a new world order, current physical laws that now lead to suffering in nature would be undone. Clearly, Moltmann's envisioning of a future world that is less regulated by deterministic principles and more by chaotic flux is connected to such hope. However, were chaotic processes rather than law-like regularities to be the order of the day in a new world, it would seem that the foundations would have

14. Wildman, "Incongruous Goodness," 291.
15. Ibid.

been laid for a world replete with developing cancers. As we have observed, open systems of life wherein that which emerges cannot be predicted by or predicated on what has gone before—such epigenetic openness and availability to novelty in biological being is the very source of cancers.

For sure, by "eternal life," nearly all Christian theologians mean more than unceasing existence, but many, if not most, imagine life without the limit of death to be a part of, if not a sine qua non for a redeemed creation. However, were we to look for models in this world for the nature of eternal being, ironically, we would find the most compelling ones in the natural progression of cancers. The most obvious example is this: the maintenance of telomere length by telomerase that is unique to cancerous life and affords cancer cells their immortality—those of Henrietta Lacks (see chapter 3) and others. And it so would appear that the structure of life today suggests that any notion of eternal life to come would be a life eternally full of cancers.

Of course, one might object that what God intends in the removal of all suffering might be a world in which our predictions based on the structures of this one, at best, do not apply or, at worst, are misleading. While he does not hold this position, Wildman summarizes a charitable appraisal of it: "a new heaven and a new earth without suffering would be so spectacular a transformation that it would have to be supernatural in character, so we should probably assume that our scientific knowledge should be ignored as irrelevant."[16] Or perhaps there is something we do not understand about cancers or about cancerous developments that would lead us to imagine that, in a redeemed world, they might become only a thing of memory.

However, our concern is less with the unlikelihood that life to come might be freed from the burden of cancer as it is with the self-contradictions in any conceivable notions that it could be. In the continuation of the citation above by Wildman, he expresses concerns that mirror ours:

> Eschatological visions of a new heaven and new earth typically involve moral and spiritual beings living in relation to one another, worshipping God, able to recognize loved ones and to remember life, able to grow and learn and change, but all this without any trace of suffering either in these blessed beings or in their natural environment. . . . Yet I cannot see how the proposals are coherent, *no matter how badly they are needed.*[17]

16. Ibid., 292.
17. Ibid.; emphasis added.

While Wildman does not specifically address whether a world to come might be spared the occurrence of cancers, we find his concern helpful for this reason: he summarizes many of our arguments that any world with entities "able to grow and learn and change" would also have to be ones containing cancers, since cancers just are processes of growth, learning, and change.

And, most importantly, we find his suggestion that hopes for a better future "might be badly needed" to be a helpful starting point for a theology of hope in a world with cancers in it. One way to understand how all these various proposals for God's redeemed world may assist us to meaningfully interpret the mystery of cancer is that they are badly needed not so much as objects of hope—that is, as descriptions of the particulars for which we are hoping—so much as they are the resources of "faithful" hope—expressions of faith in God who has something more in mind than our current world with cancers in it. Therefore, while claims for God's cancer-free future appear to be incoherent, we propose that they may rightly stir up hope in those who hear them.

From this perspective, the significance of texts from Revelation and Isaiah—and, in all theological assertions built upon them in order to portray a future world freed from natural suffering—resides not so much in their descriptions of what might come to pass, but in their promises of God's good will for us in a world that now has cancers in it, and for a promised land beyond our comprehension that will be freed from cancers.

Therefore, in the following sections we will reflect on what we mean by a hope for the future that focuses less on the details of a world freed from cancers and more on the God who promises us deliverance from the suffering that they bring about. We shall do so, first, by focusing on Gabriel Marcel's philosophy in which such hoping is considered not so much as a problem we should solve as a mystery with which we may live. And we will offer one example of lived religion that appears to exemplify this approach to hope in a world with cancer.

Hoping for Something More: Gabriel Marcel and Deanna Thompson

Earlier, we noted Marcel's distinction between problems and mysteries of living—the former being matters we might consider without involving ourselves and the latter being those that involve our innermost being. We return to that distinction here in order to develop a theology of hope in the face of cancer.

Because we believe Marcel is quite correct in claiming that "hope is a mystery and not a problem,"[18] we also hold that whenever we consider what we are hoping for apart from our "badly needing" it—this is, apart from its revealing much about the needs of our human condition—we are, in fact, not attending to the nature and impetus of our hoping. Similarly, it is misleading to regard the fulfillment of God's promise of our being delivered from cancers as a problem that we could or should solve; instead, a more fruitful approach is to accept it is a mystery to which we are bound in hope.

Marcel often distinguishes between hoping and wishing, with the latter constraining the openness of hope with its focus on particular outcomes. "The essence of hope is not 'to hope that X', but merely 'to hope.' The person who hopes does not accept the current situation as final; however, neither does she imagine or anticipate the circumstance that would deliver her from her plight, rather she merely hopes for deliverance.[19]

While what Marcel here describes may sound more like resignation to whatever comes our way rather than an expectation for deliverance from current trouble, hope is not a passive waiting but an active searching out and looking forward, an awaiting something new and something better. Hope is not acceptance of our current circumstances as all that God has to offer. Rather, hope is directed toward God's good intents and, most appropriately, toward God in Godself. "Hope consists in asserting that there is at the heart of being, beyond all data, beyond all inventories and all calculations, a mysterious principle which is in *connivance with me*, which cannot but will that which I will, if what I will deserves to be willed and is, in fact, willed by the whole of my being."[20]

Simply put, our hoping is always constituted by a longing for God and the benefits of communion with God. And as a turning to this Eternal Thou, our hope is always connected with the many finite thous—those persons around us—as part of the anticipated salvation. "There can be no hope that does not constitute itself through a 'we' and for a 'we.' I would be tempted to say that all hope is at the bottom choral."[21]

18. Marcel, *Homo Viator*, 35.

19. Marcel, *The Philosophy of Existentialism*, 28.

20. Ibid.; emphasis added.

21. Marcel, *Homo Viator*, 143.

Accordingly, a person who hopes is less like one who demands to know precisely how something good will occur and more like "the inventor or the discoverer who says, 'There must be a way' and who adds: 'I am going to find it.' She who hopes says simply: 'It will be found.'"[22] To be sure, what Marcel calls "established experience" (what we see and have always seen around us) may suggest that all will be as it has been, that added time will add nothing new, that nothing new will emerge—to say it simply, that nothing more awaits us. However, when we hope, we hope for something more.

We turn now to some reflections by Deanna Thompson, a Lutheran theologian who has focused on questions of God and human suffering in Luther's thought, because we find her thoughts to be illustrative of such hoping for something more. In summarizing the shape of her recent years, Thompson writes, "People used to marvel—sometimes with admiration, sometimes with envy—at my near-perfect life."[23] Given these experiences, Thompson reports that she believed she could scarcely "hope for more." And even "some annoying back pain" and a subsequent MRI did not seem likely to interfere with this perfect world, since Thompson had been told, "One in a thousand chances it's cancer."[24]

But breast cancer it was, the most advanced stage possible. In response to her cancer, Thompson has reflected in a variety of ways including journal and online articles, and in her recently published cancer memoir, *Hoping for More, Having Cancer, Talking Faith, and Accepting Grace*, about her life, about the Christian life, about cancer—and about hope. "What living in hope does mean is that I am learning to trust that grace is sufficient for today, for tomorrow, and beyond. And that whatever happens, I know that grace will continue to accompany me on the rest of my journey through this life and even into the next."[25] To our ears, Thompson here is articulating a hope that resonates with that proposed by Marcel—trust in the goodness of God whatever comes. That is, her hope is not dependent on the occurrence of a pre-designated outcome.

And, also consonant with Marcel's concept of hope, Thompson does hope for something more—that is, something other than her life now with cancer. Thompson does not know exactly what might be this something that is more than what is now, but she trusts that beyond her own suffering

22. Marcel, *The Philosophy of Existentialism*, 51–52.

23. Thompson, *Hoping for More*, 1.

24. Ibid., 5, 9.

25. Ibid., 144.

and all suffering, something more will come her way. "For all of us who struggle to trust in these promises—even in the midst of deadly conditions—hearing that there's more than just this terminal diagnosis or that life-shattering earthquake offers a word of hope. That the suffering of this world isn't the final word is an essential part of the gospel's good news."[26]

Here Thompson articulates a tension between living with the reality of this world and hearing the promise of another one. As she does, she also observes that many feminist theologians like herself have been reluctant to speak in much detail—or even at all—about some other reality, because doing so might divert from grappling with the sufferings and injustices of this one. And Thompson indicates other reasons for her having hesitated to focus on hoping for something more that we recognize as related to our concerns noted earlier about whether there could ever be coherent descriptions of a cancer-free existence:

> While Christian faith talks of heavenly feasts and bodily resurrection, many of us struggle with how to set these claims alongside the science of decomposing flesh or suspicions regarding consciousness beyond the grave. In light of these tensions that govern contemporary understandings of materiality and death, what should theologians be saying about our future life with God?[27]

We, too, have noted some of these limits, and also the struggle to depict any kind of biological being, both now and in all times, without the enduring presence of cancers.

Immediately following the citation above, Thompson continues, "I don't pretend to have adequate answers to these questions."[28] Nor do we, and we suggest that there may be none since they appear to reduce the mystery of cancer to a problem—a process that may be helpful to the accumulation of scientific knowledge about treating cancer but may not be for faithful understandings of God's promise for a cancer-free future.

Thompson does not so much offer an answer but rather describes ways she has addressed these questions through a community of inquiry that joins her in grappling with them. She tells that, in her teaching of undergraduates, she decided not to keep her classroom conversation "cancer free." Accordingly:

26. Ibid., 145.
27. Ibid., 146.
28. Ibid.

One student suggested that Christian faith is ultimately a kind of wager. In faith Christians wager that God accompanies us in our suffering and that through Christ, God promises that sin, death, and destruction will not triumph in the end. For some of my students, such a wager was too big a gamble. For others, it's an outrageous claim lacking sufficient evidence. But for still others, they—like me—were working to stake their lives on it.[29]

In hearing this account, we are reminded of a remark by a cancer researcher colleague in response to our work on cancer and evolution:

Science argues on the basis of evidence and, on those grounds, the warrant for hope in a world of evolution is not strong. From the findings of evolution, you've got millions of suffering and extinct species on the one hand, and if you've got faith, you've got only one resurrected person in Jesus. The evidence does lend much weight to hope. But, still, it might be the truth and worth putting one's money on.

Thompson's story is a rich one, so rich that we do not wish to confine it to an analysis of how it may exemplify certain principles of Marcel's philosophy of hope. Thus, we will return to her reflections later, but here we note how Marcel and Thompson are alike in describing hope as a trust that we will be granted deliverance by God even when no evidence is available for such a hope.

Still, we are led to ask: might there be any sources of hope in the "established evidence" around us—in current cancer facts—that might give us hope that God will provide "deliverance"?

God in Connivance with Us: Sources of Hope in Our World of Cancers

"In hoping, I do not create in the strict sense of the word, but I appeal to the existence of a certain power in the world, or rather to the actual resources at the disposal of this creative power."[30]

In the previous chapter, we noted that, because of chance, cancers appear to be a statistical inevitability in this world. We also observed that many particular instances of cancer display a juggernaut quality as the odds of

29. Ibid., 75.
30. Marcel, *Homo Viator*, 52.

their developing into a deadly life-force within their host increases over time. And in this chapter we have noted that a close reading of cancer science strongly makes it difficult to depict how it would not be present in all life realms—both now and in any time that is to come.

But are there already any sources of hope about the occurrences of cancer in this world as it now is? By such sources of hope, we mean those facts about the disease that, while they cannot prove that God, in Marcel's words, is in "connivance with us," may be received in faith as indicators or pointers that God is inclined to be so? Here is another way to ask this question: are there any facts about cancer shown us in the science of the disease that we might see as signs of hope in a world with cancers in them?

We think that there are many such cancers facts that, in faith, we may understand to be sources of hope that God has something more in mind than this world with cancers in it. These facts do not so much demonstrate as suggest that God is our help in this time and may be our hope in times to come. These are the facts: (1) not all genetic mutations that might initiate cancers will always do so; (2) some cells with mutations that do begin to develop into true cancers will not necessarily succeed in doing so; (3) before the events referred to in (1) and (2) might occur, many exposures to carcinogens may be avoided and/or eliminated—thereby removing the initiation of many cancers. We start with the first.

At the startling rate of more than 30,000 incidents per day, every cell in our bodies suffers myriad types of DNA damage. Owing to our many and redundant DNA repair mechanisms, the vast majority of these injuries are repaired effectively and without alteration. Over the years, then, all cells accumulate random mutations, some of which inevitably alter cell fate by disabling genes that perform vital functions necessary to cell homeostasis ... or as protectors of this homeostasis; or by reactivating long-silent genes whose missions were fulfilled during development *in utero*, and whose reinvigoration may throw the formerly well-behaved cell into a frenzy of unregulated cell division.

While cancers develop from random mutations of DNA, the occurrence of any one of these mutations does not mean that a cancer will necessarily result. As noted, many genetic hits are required and often must occur in a particular sequence in order to promote oncogenesis. If they do not, the abnormal progression will terminate early in the otherwise long developmental process that leads to cancer. By chance, therefore, a cell may never acquire the particular mutational load necessary for conversion to malignancy.

Yet a second source of hoping may be extracted from the following fact about cancer: even if a cell does accumulate the necessary genetic alterations to develop into a true cancer, it still may not succeed in doing so. There are many examples of this. For instance, we have long known that immunosuppression greatly increases the risk for developing cancer—which is why Kaposi's sarcoma, an exceedingly rare cancer, is a common ailment among persons with HIV infection. Therefore, it is abundantly clear that our immune system is primed to wipe out incipient cancer cells and does so with great efficiency. And p53, the quintessential tumor suppressor and guardian of our genome, enforces the destruction of abnormal and genetically unstable cells (apoptosis) before they can become fully malignant. Furthermore, even among cancers that achieve the potential for malignant spread, only a few will succeed in doing so. It is estimated that only one in a million will survive the journey through the bloodstream to colonize distant sites.

There is an important but often-overlooked implication to this fact that even with an initial genetic loading that predicts a likely development of a cancer, a cancer still may not develop. The implication is that genes are not mechanical destiny. To be sure, for certain diseases a single genetic mishap is all it takes for them to arise. Some examples are: sickle-cell anemia, which is a defect in the hemoglobin molecule that transports oxygen from the lungs to the tissues, or cystic fibrosis (CF) in which the mutated CF gene cannot maintain the thin watery mucus layer that enables proper clearance of pathogens and particles from lungs. However, with the exception of certain rare childhood leukemias, cancer is not a single-gene disease—and these are the exceptions that prove a general rule of oncological science that has bearings for theological study and religious life informed by such inquiry.

For example, after describing various genetic factors in the origins of cancers, The Evangelical Lutheran Church in America in its Social Statement on Genetics observed, "There will be those who mistakenly believe that genes alone determine the destiny of . . . the world, and who, accordingly, approach life with a kind of fatalism."[31] We concur that such an approach is a mistake. The science of cancer genetics does not provide data to support despair but, in the situations noted above, to offer hope by demonstrating that not all cancerous genotypes—mutations and abnormalities of DNA—will result in cancers.

31. Evangelical Lutheran Church in America, "A Social Statement," 33.

So, we have noted two facts about cancer basic science that may be sources of hope: not all mutations that might lead to cancerous development will do so and even those cells that do begin to do so may stop or be stopped somewhere in their tracks. There is yet another source of hope in a world of cancers: there is no necessity for many of the events that might start a cancerous process to take place. Rather, many of these carcinogens—agents and exposures that initiate cancers—may be avoided or eliminated.

As we have noted, there are many sources for genetic damage. To be sure, all cells are constantly suffering DNA damage caused by their own internal processes at the rate of approximately 30,000 events per day. However, added to this intrinsic background rate of mutation are exposures to such external agents as UV radiation, tobacco, and alcohol, which can heap on far higher rates of mutation in the affected tissues.

The good news is that many of these external exposures can be controlled or eliminated. Perhaps the most obvious are those cancers for whose occurrence somewhere between a medium (e.g., bladder and head and neck) to very high percentage (e.g., lung) may be attributed to tobacco use. Furthermore, direct and downstream smoking account for over 20 percent of cancers deaths worldwide, and in developed/high-resource countries, for over one-third of those deaths.[32] Accordingly, cancer control researchers and public agencies direct an enormous amount of dollars, time, and energy into eliminating a leading source of cancer suffering and cancer death.

There are other controllable carcinogens, not all of which we can consider here, but one is worth highlighting because of its recent rise in public awareness and because it is a dream come true for many cancer researchers—a vaccine. Without the occurrence of HPV infections, there would be nearly no cervical cancers. Currently, cervical cancer is the second most common cancer in women around the world.[33] However, the recent development of a vaccine that may remove the nearly necessary cause of this cancer means that it is reasonable to hope that, someday, it might never exist.

We list these two causes of cancers, tobacco use and HPV infections, as exemplary of the many cancers that need not occur as frequently as they now do. Both illustrate how the incidence of cancers that occur may be

---

32. Boyle and Levin, eds., *The World Cancer Report 2008*, 110.

33. See ibid., 418: "Epidemiological studies have shown that the human papillomavirus (HPV) is the central cause of cervical cancer, WCR and the prevalence of HPV in cervical cancer has been shown to be close to 100%." See also Franco et al., "Epidemiologic Evidence and Human Papillomavirus."

changed. There are, to use Marcel's language, "actual resources at the dis-posal" of the creative power of God that we, even with our strategizing to prevent the occurrences of these and other cancers, do not so much create as receive and interpret as signs of the mystery that God is in connivance with us in ways to avoid the occurrence of cancers.

In addition to the ways in which these features of cancerous develop-ment may be interpreted and received as sources of hope in God and God's goodness, there is another that demands careful consideration: sometimes a change for the better in the suffering brought on by cancers may be as-sisted by our very hoping for such change.

A Leap in the Dark: Changing Cancer by Hoping that Cancer Can Be Changed

> Let us suppose that I develop some incurable illness and that my condition shows no improvement. It may be that I say of myself, "I cannot be cured." . . . [I]t seems as though I decide and defy any real or possible contradictions. . . . In this way, I pronounce my own sentence . . . Is there not now every chance that, discouraged by this sentence, I will feel obliged to confirm it? So it comes about that, far from merely foreseeing my own destiny, I shall really have precipitated it.[34]

In reflecting on hope, Marcel also considered its opposite—despair, or ca-pitulation to fate. For Marcel, capitulation is not so much acceptance of alleged inevitabilities, but a process of "going to pieces" (in the precise sense of losing one's personal integrity) and consequent "disarming of one-self" before them. And, as evident in the above citation, Marcel understood such "anticipation of destruction" might be a self-fulfilling prophecy. By con-trast, when we hope, we may create new realities in the world: "in so far as I hope, I detach myself from this inner determinism. . . . [H]ope has the power of making things fluid."[35]

Before Marcel, the pragmatist philosopher William James proposed some very similar notions about the power of beliefs to create new and bet-ter realities. "There are then cases where a fact cannot come at all unless a preliminary faith exists that it will do so.[36] For James, the act of believing

34. Marcel, *Homo Viator*, 37.
35. Ibid., 41.
36. James, *The Will to Believe*, 85.

(and he conceived of beliefs more as verbs/activities rather than as nouns/ entities) can and, sometimes, does effect situations, and can thereby bring new facts into the world. And the contrapositive also holds: not believing that something may come about may actually contribute its non-occurrence.

As an example of that, James related an incident when two armed bandits on a packed train successfully robbed all its passengers, in part, because no single passenger believed anyone else onboard would join him or her in resisting them. On the other hand, believing may contribute to the creation of new realities—for example, an athlete's determination to break a long-established performance record may actually assist in his doing so. Another illustration from James: a person who finds herself at a mountainous precipice and who must attempt to jump it because she cannot reverse her course may only succeed in her leap if she believes that she might succeed and might fail if she believes that she cannot. "In all important transactions of life we have to take a leap in the dark."[37]

We believe that analogous situations exist for some persons with cancer: some may actually succeed in changing aspects of their cancers because they hope they can do so. The following example, shared with us by the brother of one of our colleagues, illustrates this fact. It was not until this colleague's brother, who knew that he was suffering with an often fatal type of brain cancer, had first hoped that he might be cured of his cancer that he, subsequently, was able to be cured of it. How so? Because it was not until he had hoped his disease might be cured that he then sought out the recommended medical treatment that, effectively, did cure it. Sometimes hoping for a diminution to the suffering of cancers may contribute to a hoped-for decrease—because such hoping may spur persons to seek out remedies that may help.

Here, we caution our readers by calling attention to the fact that believing or hoping alone for good results from medical treatments never guarantees that better times are ahead. Beyond the personal considerations of the various costs—financial, personal or others sorts—involved in most medical treatment, there remains the enduring fact upon which we focused in the previous chapter and which we highlight here: *some particular cases of cancers appear to be refractory to all interventions.* Perhaps even more importantly, some persons who are dying from and also have accepted that they will die from cancer may still report that they are dying with some kind of hope. For example, some hospice patients who were anticipating

37. Ibid., 87.

their deaths have shared that they still experience hope by "recollecting themselves"—that is, by resisting a "going to pieces" before the inevitability of their death.[38]

On the other hand, we do believe that sometimes hoping for change in cancers may truly be what James called "living options" for those who hold them—that is, responses to opportunities that may produce better realities even when the "established evidence" does not suggest that betterment is likely to occur. In *The Emperor of All Maladies*, Mukherjee relates the story of Barbara Bradfield who, in 1990, had been clearly informed by her physicians—and therefore had come to believe as certain—that she would die from her recently diagnosed breast cancer. "I was at the end of my road and I had accepted what seemed inevitable."[39] Consequently, it took more than one call from the cancer researcher, Dennis Slamon, to convince her to enroll in a clinical trial for his then newly minted and now widely administered drug, Herceptin, that did, in fact, save her life. "For Bradford, Slamon's second phone call was an omen that was not missed; something in that conversation pierced through a shield that she had drawn around herself."[40] Perhaps for not all important matters, but, certainly for some, it is necessary to take a leap in the dark.

The story above also illustrates another practical bearing of hope in a world with cancers: the envisioning and consequent development of more effective treatments for those with the disease. To be sure, as we have carefully noted in the previous chapter, "inevitability" does characterize a haunting quality of both the pervasiveness of cancers throughout the world and of an unstoppable feature of this disease in certain individual cases. Yet, Sui Hang, who earlier strongly emphasized the "necessity of cancers," does not despair:

> [T]he expression 'inevitability' of cancer' . . . only shall alert us of how the process of tumorigenesis is deeply linked to our very existence as complex, evolved and developing organisms. It shall not stifle the hope to find a way to avert the self-perpetuating, tragic consequences of accidental developmental errors. Thus, this long, winding journey offers many points for modulation by lifestyle and intervention with drugs.[41]

38. Benzein et al., "The Meaning of the Lived Experience of Hope," 123. The authors turn to Marcel to describe such *"living in hope,* that is reconciliation with and comfort with life and death."

39. Mukherjee, *The Emperor of All Maladies,* 420.

40. Ibid.

41. Huang, "On the Intrinsic Inevitability of Cancer," 196.

There is, then, much to hope for in this world with cancers. Many responses to cancers that were once barely imaginable and hardly conceivable—not only vaccines but also targeted therapies like that which Bradford received because Slamon hoped for and then conceived of it—are not only possible, but, now, are quite real.

And there is more to hope for. In a later chapter, we will discuss how we increasingly have the ability to cut into the evolutionary flow of many cancers and thereby divert their course. In doing so, we will consider how, amidst the chance and necessity of cancer, we may produce, and increasingly are producing, better scientific understandings of and, consequently, treatments for cancer—in part, because we have hoped that such understandings and treatments were possible.

Conclusion: Acceptance and Hope as Two Wise Responses

In considering the aptness of the phrase, "the very fiber of our being," to describe cancer, we noted in chapter 1 that, while both persons employed that same phrase, Saint Peregrine Laziosi appeared to respond to cancer in one way, and Walter Wangerin in another.[42] Simplified, the response of the former, since he perceived cancer to be a threat to that fiber, is hope, while that of the latter, who views it as being of the same fiber as the rest of himself, is acceptance.

Of course, this simplification is just that—an overview that omits complexities, thereby passing over the elements of acceptance present in Peregrine's prayers to God, and Wangerin's hope that is founded on Christ's victory over death. Similarly, elements of hope may be discerned in the theological positions outlined in the previous chapter and those of acceptance in this one. Thus, Karl Peters experienced a hope beyond death even as his wife died from cancer. And Ted Peters continues to speak of the goodness of creation as God continues to create a hoped for future. This mixture of elements from both these religious positions mirrors the theologies of not only Saint Peregrine and Walter Wangerin, but also the lived religion of millions of other persons with cancer who live in both acceptance and hope.

Still, in our analyses of these two perspectives, we have detected some clear differences between them with the result that, considered in sum, each appears to offer a distinctly faithful understanding and wise

42. See pages 13–15.

response. The first position strongly holds that, in all creation, there can be "no exclusion of suffering" in God's creation because that creation is one in which cancers inevitably are a part of it. Accepting this means not only a "letting go" before the world and God, but also a turning toward the world with its sufferings and to the God who may empower us to bear them. And, though the perspective that we have considered in this chapter does not exclude this first one, this second perspective in all its variations—whether or not they include a transformed world in a time to come—does propose something more: that God will deliver us from the sufferings brought on by cancers.

How may we assess these two positions for an evolutionary theology of cancer? We begin by offering what we intend as a critical appreciation for those faithful perspectives for which, at the start of this chapter, we offered our most critical remarks: theologies of hope that attempt to depict a time to come freed from all cancers. We understand the impetus for these particular eschatological perspectives to have many sources that we not only respect but also heartily endorse. One is the conviction that the God who once created and ordered this good world both still does so and will continue to do so in order that all of God's good purposes for it may be realized. In hoping for a better world, this position takes seriously the ills of this world and discerns in current times remedies for some of them that foreshadow the removal of all ills.

Another source for our positive appraisal is found in the sentiments by Robert John Russell that we noted earlier and that are worth revisiting: the redemption of creation hopes to involve "the curing of disease and the overcoming of death," including diseases of multi-cellular life.[43] What warrant might Russell and the rest of us have for hoping for so much? Because, in faith, we may hope that God is Lord of not only our religious experiences of accepting and hoping, but of far more and much vaster things: of all that is in human history and in the natural order, including cancers.

Therefore, while we believe that an evolutionary theology of cancer must contain a consideration of the "inevitability of cancers," we also believe that it must somehow incorporate the truth of claims like that of Ted Peters, that "God has promised that death is going to be replaced by resurrection, and suffering will be no more."[44] Therefore, an evolutionary theology of cancer will maintain certain truths of both these faithful understandings.

43. Russell, "The Groaning of Creation," 139–40.
44. Peters and Hewlett, *Evolution from Creation to New Creation*, 158.

In doing so, an evolutionary theology of cancer will also incorporate their wise responses that we must both accept that we live in a world of cancers and also hope for something more.

Already in our discussions of this chapter, we have hinted how we may begin to reconcile these theological understandings and wise responses. In our review of certain cancer facts—that many cancers may not be initiated that might have been, that many of these initiated cancers will not develop deadly abilities, and that many sources of oncogenesis itself may be eliminated or avoided—we have suggested that, accordingly, God may be confessed as having something more in mind for this world than the ways cancer is now present in it. Also, by taking a "leap in the dark," our hoping itself may introduce new and better facts into this world. To be sure, even with such hoping, certain features of cancers that produce suffering or death may remain intact, but sometimes hoping may give birth to actions that may alter some of them. Sometimes, the very process of hoping may modify certain "inevitabilities" of cancer.

For an evolutionary theology of cancer, we also note another source for reconciling these two differing faithful understandings with their consequentially different wise responses. That is this: along with their differences, they are united in believing God to be the source of their responses of acceptance and hope. For it is God who enables us to accept the world as it is with its cancers. And it is God who creates in us the hope for something more than this world with cancers in it. Furthermore, both propose that God is continuously creating to bring good to this world through the same evolutionary processes of chance and necessity that also bring cancers to it. And both describe God's work through these evolutionary processes as a way in which divine love for the world is at work.

Accordingly, in the following chapter, we will turn our attention to both scientific and theological understandings of the concepts of chance and necessity in order to consider how the divine may be discerned amidst the evolutionary chance and necessity of cancers. In doing so, we shall propose that it is the love of God for this world as it is and as it shall be that enables us to both accept what is inevitable about cancers and also to hope for more. And we will offer a schema for how the love of God may be discerned in, with, and under the chance and necessity of cancers.

Chapter 6

Chance, Necessity, Love:
A Theology of Cancer

I n the previous chapters, we have examined two faithful understandings
of cancer. One is that God has created a world in which various forms of
suffering, including cancers, are inevitable. The other is that God intends to
provide us deliverance from cancers and the sufferings they may bring with
them. Each of these faithful understandings suggests a concomitantly wise
response to existence of cancers. The first, acceptance, is to face our finitude
and consequent forms of suffering. The second, hope, is to anticipate that
changes in such suffering for the better may come about, and through such
hoping sometimes to even help changes occur.

In our review of these theological positions, we have also observed
that, even with their differences, both share an appreciation for the ways
that cancers come into being through the processes of evolutionary chance
and necessity. In this chapter, we will continue to develop our evolutionary
theology of cancer first by examining the ways that three important thinkers have grappled with the principles of evolutionary chance and necessity
themselves and then by considering the implications of their having done
so for understanding the love of God in a world containing the chance and
necessity of cancer. This analysis will enable us to propose a theology of the
love of God in, with, and under the chance and necessity of cancers.

Now we turn to the perspectives of Jacques Monod, Arthur Peacocke,
and Charles Sanders Peirce on evolutionary phenomena. These three

thinkers will be the primary interlocutors for our inquiry into an evolutionary theology of cancer both in this chapter and in our conclusion.

Three Perspectives on Chance, Necessity, and Cancer

"Chance as Free and Blind": Jacques Monod

When he published in 1970 a short treatise entitled *Chance and Necessity: An Essay on the Natural Philosophy of Modern Biology*, Jacques Monod had long been renowned among his fellow researchers in molecular biology. Monod's reception, along with François Jacob and André Lwoff, of the Nobel Prize five years earlier "for their discoveries concerning genetic control of enzyme and virus synthesis" had brought him broad public recognition and even prestige, especially in France.[1] Thus, during the pitched student-police battles in Paris during the spring of 1968, the name of Monod was invoked by authorities as a leading citizen of the Republic in an attempt to bring calm to the capital.

But even on the basis of Monod's scientific achievements and social standing, no one could have imagined the earthquake that the publication of his little work would cause throughout the world. At just under 200 pages, much of it summarized then current findings in biochemical research and their evolutionary implications with a detail that, according to one reviewer, rendered comprehension by most general readers "a little unrealistic."[2] Still, while many who picked up the book struggled to grasp its resume of evolutionary biology, almost all were impressed—some positively, some not—with what Monod himself claimed to be the major implication of that science: life arises, not out of any comprehensive plan or according to any comprehensible order, but out of chance which:

> alone is at the source of every innovation, of all creation in the biosphere. Pure chance, absolutely free but blind, at the very root of the stupendous edifice of evolution edifice of evolution: today this central concept of modern biology.[3]

While the title of Monod's book was *Chance and Necessity*, the text itself focuses mostly on the former evolutionary dynamism, and less on

1. "Jacques Monod—Facts."
2. Steiner, "Chance and Necessity," 5.
3. Monod, *Chance and Necessity*, 112–13.

the latter. To be sure, necessary or law-like regularities of natural selection govern the outcomes of chance, but what those laws direct throughout evolution comes about from no necessary causes and for no purposes. Consequently, "the ancient covenant is in pieces; man knows at last that he is alone in the universe's unfeeling immensity, out of which he emerged only by chance. His destiny is nowhere spelled out, nor is his duty. The kingdom above or the darkness below; it is for him to choose."[4]

In the preface to *Chance and Necessity*, Monod cites a portion from Albert Camus' seminal short work, *The Myth of Sisyphus*—and, throughout his own work, Monod embraced a view of the human condition connected to Camus and other existentialist philosophers of the mid- to late twentieth century.[5] As a result, some have linked Monod to, or seen him as the prototype for the twenty-first century's spate of scientific scoffers of religion. However, Monod was not, like many current scientific atheists, so much a cultured despiser of religion as one who, with some heaviness of heart like Camus, forswore not only theological understandings of nature but all attempts to detect any purpose for it. Furthermore, Monod was descended from a long line of Huguenots, and it is arguable that a trace Stoicism sometimes at work in that Calvinist tradition may have been operative in his call to sternly face the world as it is—or, at least, as he understood it.[6] Whether or not Monod did appropriate this tradition for his own philosophy of human being in the face of chance and necessity, he clearly did propose that the world is governed, not by inscrutable providence, but by austere fate. And he understood there to be a confluence between his biological research and Camus' thought: "each of science's conquests is a victory of the absurd."[7]

Descended from privilege, Monod both took advantage of many opportunities that came his way and sought out some for himself within the scientific community in order to focus on the origins of life, with a particular emphasis on how genetic information was passed along, since genes, themselves, are inert. Working with Francois Jacob, he explained the mechanisms by which the text stacked within the genetic library actually instructs molecular activities—that is, the way in which genetic information

4. Ibid., 180.

5. See Carrol, *Brave Genius*.

6. Stanier, "Obituary." "Jacques Monod accordingly had a Calvinist and puritan family background on the maternal as well as the paternal side" (1). "Although separated by at least one generation from Protestant religion, Monod was imbued with the sternest and most pitiless version of the Protestant ethos: at heart, he remained a Calvinist" (11).

7. Monod, *Lecon inaugurale*, 27.

actually informs. Consequently, Monod's remark, "I have discovered the second secret of life," is only mildly hyperbolic. And while their studies did not focus on cancer, Monod and his colleague did not miss the importance of their findings for its origins in genetic mishaps: "malignancy is adequately described as a breakdown of one or several growth controlling systems, and the genetic origin of this breakdown can hardly be doubted."[8]

Along with his successes, Monod's life was also one of struggle. During the Second World War, he remained in Paris where he assumed major leadership in the underground resistance. And though his name was invoked in order to bring peace during the 1968 uprising in Paris, he received a cold shoulder at a gathering of students on whose behalf he interceded. There is a striking, close-up photo of Monod several days afterwards as he, carefully holding the hand of a blinded student and escorting her away from the street fighting, looks forward longingly while an accompanying Red Cross worker beckons for assistance. An epitome of Monod's lifelong striving for a better world may be found in his final words that, as he lay dying of leukemia, he whispered to his brother, "Je cherche à comprendre," "I am trying to understand."[9]

While Monod's studies did not concentrate on cancer, the effects of his "trying to understand" for cancer studies continue to transcend his death. Thus, in Paris today, major research on cancer is conducted at the Institut Jacques Monod. Furthermore, Monod's reflections on chance and necessity continue to bear much fruit in cancer biology as evidenced in the following selection of recent works in that field. Monod's groundbreaking work on messenger RNA is noted in a 2011 article, "The Biological and Therapeutic Relevance of mRNA Translation in Cancer."[10] In "Models of Experimental Evolution: The Role of Genetic Chance and Selective Necessity," the authors identify many selective forces in the midst of chance genetic mutations at work in the development of cancers.[11] In "Chance or Necessity? Insertional Mutagenesis in Gene Therapy and Its Consequences," Monod's landmark book is cited and then its categories employed to suggest ways to prevent leukemias that may result from therapeutic gene insertions.[12] Again, his legacy is evident in an assessment of the relationship between of one's

8. Jacob and Monod, "Genetic Regulatory Mechanisms," 354.

9. Judson, *The Eighth Day*, 616.

10. Blagden and Willis, "The Biological and Therapeutic Relevance."

11. Wahl and Krakauer, "Models of Experimental Evolution."

12. Baum et al., "Chance or Necessity?"

occupation and exposure to carcinogens in "Lung Cancer among Silica-Exposed Workers: The Quest for Truth between Chance and Necessity."[13] And Monod's work informed Sui Huang's essay, "Cancer as Developmental Disease: Chance and Necessity in Networks Dynamics During Somatic Evolution of Cancer Cells" that was foundational for his previously noted work on the inevitability of cancers.[14]

The above list does not exhaust the practical bearings of Monod's reflections for contemporary cancer science but we draw to a close our testimony to their effects by turning to the article, "Chance and Necessity in Arthur Peacocke's Scientific Work," by Gayle Woloschak, a cancer researcher and also Associate Director of the Zygon Center for Religion and Science.[15] Having considered her conclusions, we will explore Peacocke's own engagement with Monod as this biologist and religious thinker tried to understand the role of chance and necessity in various evolutionary phenomena, including cancers. As we will see, Peacocke's lifelong conversation with Monod contributed to the field of religion and science and contributes to our evolutionary theology of cancer.

Creation in, with, and under Chance and Necessity: Arthur Peacocke

In her review of Peacocke's scientific work, Woloschak proposes that his early scientific study of mutagenesis—a source of cancers—launched his lifelong commitment to studies in science and religion. An accomplished molecular biologist, Peacocke made significant and enduring discoveries about a variety of DNA functions, and, in particular, the ways in which radiation may alter those processes.

While it is a matter of chance whether or not a mutation will result from any single exposure to radiation, the effects following all mutations that happen to occur are predictable. These "deterministic" outcomes suggested first to Peacocke, and, in time, to many others, that more than "blind chance" was at work not only in the effects of mutagenesis but throughout all evolutionary events:

13. Cocco et al., "Lung Cancer."

14. Huang, "Cancer as Developmental Disease"; "On the Intrinsic Inevitability of Cancer."

15. Woloschak, "Chance and Necessity."

Nature and life processes involve a combination of chance occurrences and processes that are mediated by necessity (or are deterministic in nature). For example, by necessity, a change in climate to a colder environment will select for a certain set of survival features that are predictable—thicker fur over thinner hair, longer sleep cycle over shorter sleep cycle, slower metabolism over faster metabolism, etc. Because these sets of . . . features can be predicted from a set of known parameters, they are deterministic or driven by necessity.[16]

What did Peacocke mean by chance and necessity? And why did he think that Monod's explanations of their functions in nature were inadequate?

First, chance: Peacocke understood there to be two meanings. Sometimes, the term *chance* refers to the way in which some events cannot be predicted to result from any cause or set of causes. In other words (ours), all physical occurrences have one or more proximate or distant causes—the fall of a Newtonian apple may involve the force of the wind, the ripeness of the fruit, and always includes gravity—but for some events, the attribution of clear and distinct causal factors to the production of specified results is meaningless. Peacocke employs the familiar case of coin tossing as an example. A number of factors cause each toss to turn up heads or tails, but these factors are so many and their effects are so unpredictable that we may say that the results of these factors are brought on by chance.

The second meaning of chance applies to those events that occur, not for any reason, but by accident—that is, when two or more things meet, intersect, collide, or overlap that do not have to so. "Suppose that when you leave the building in which you are reading these pages, as you step onto the pavement you are struck on the head by a hammer dropped by a man repairing the roof. . . . In ordinary parlance we would say it was due to 'pure chance.'"[17]

Peacocke employs both of these meanings to explain findings from his early cancer research on the processes by which radiation may cause genetic mutations. One process is the "interplay" between the genes of an organism and particular environmental pressures on them. "These two causal chains are entirely independent, and it is in the second sense of chance that Monod is correct in saying that evolution depends on chance."[18] The other sense

16. Ibid., 83
17. Peacocke, "Chance and the Life Game," 304.
18. Peacocke, "Chance and Law," 126.

of chance—that of unpredictability—also applies "since, in most cases we are not now in a position to specify all the factors which led to the mutated organisms being selected and, even less, the mechanism by which mutation was induced in the first place."[19]

While chance is at work in the biological world, so also is "necessity" or "law." By both of these terms, Peacocke meant the principles that govern events in the world that we may predict will occur and that we may assert are bound to occur. These directive dynamisms include "the fundamental physical constants, the fundamental particles as well as the physical laws of the interrelation of matter, energy, space, and time and of other physical features of the universe."[20]

From his observations that "laws arise that do structure and control events in the world," Peacocke concluded, "there is no reason why the randomness of molecular events in relation to biological consequence has to be given the significant metaphysical status that Monod attributed to it."[21] Here, Peacocke contended with Monod not as a metaphysician, but as a scientist in arguing that principles of necessity (or law) are at work in the world: "as we already have seen in the behavior of matter on a larger scale, many regularities, which have been raised to the level of being describable as 'laws,' arise from the combined effect of random microscopic events which constitute the macroscopic."[22]

Throughout his career, Peacocke argued for the ways in which chance and necessity together drive evolutionary developments:

> From the interaction of genetic mutations and natural selection, from the role of so-called chance events, in the emergence and development of life, many (as we saw) who have reflected on the processes of biological evolution have concluded that they are "due to chance" and therefore of no significance for man's understanding of the universe and of his place in it. These studies demonstrate that the interplay of chance and law is in fact creative, for it is the combination of the two which allows new forms to emerge and evolve.[23]

Over time, Peacocke's views on the importance of law-like regularities in evolutionary phenomena have found much resonance. In his review

19. Peacocke, "Chance and the Life Game," 306.

20. Ibid., 320–21.

21. Peacocke, "Welcoming the 'Disguised Friend,'" 476.

22. Peacocke, "Chance and the Life Game," 307.

23. Ibid., 314.

of Monod's book and of scientific findings since its publication thirty-five years earlier, the eminent biologist Christian de Duve concludes, "less chance, more necessity. Such, in a nutshell, is the message emerging so far from the preceding overview. Squeezed between deterministic chemistry and optimizing selection, contingency has enjoyed less leeway than was believed by Monod."[24] The also renowned molecular biologist Francis Ayala similarly observes, "The theory of evolution manifests chance and necessity jointly intwined in the stuff of life; randomness and determinism interlocked in a natural process that has spurted the most complex, diverse, and beautiful entities in the universe."[25]

As a scientist, Peacocke discerned many ways in which life continued to evolve through the interplay of chance and necessity. From his study of theology, he concluded that God created and sustained through these same evolutionary processes: "this combination for a theist, can only be regarded as an aspect of the God-endowed features of the world. . . . God is the ultimate ground and source of both law ('necessity') and "chance."[26] In bringing life into the world, God acts like a musical composer who extemporizes "a fugue to creation [of] the world *through* what we call 'chance' operating within the created order, each stage of which constitutes the launching pad for the next."[27] That is, Peacocke proposed that God's acts of creation are kenotic, "whereby *God suffers in, with and under the creative processes of the world* with their costly, open-ended unfolding in time."[28]

In his early theological reflections, Peacocke proposed, therefore, that God is present in the fugal compositions of creation much the way a composer is present in performances of his/her works. In the decades that followed, Peacocke became a leader in a religion/science scholarship burgeoning with writings on evolution, chance, and necessity. As more proposals, each with its own melodic line, were put forward, Peacocke conducted himself much like a composer of fugues by harmoniously weaving his own line of thought into the mix. And as Peacocke was dying from cancer, the compliment was returned by a gathering of theologians who invited him to summarize his life's work on many matters including "natural evil" or the suffering brought on by creation: "when faced with this ubiquity

24. De Duve, "Thoughts of a Senior Scientist," 3156.
25. Ayala, "Chance and Necessity," 238.
26. Peacocke "Welcoming the 'Disguised Friend,'" 477.
27. Ibid.
28. Peacocke, *Theology for a Scientific Age*, 126.

of pain, suffering, and death in the evolution of the living world, we are impelled to infer that God, to be anything like the God who *is* Love—must be understood to be suffering in, with, and under the creative processes of the world."[29] About Peacocke's offering to this collective, the editor of their responses wrote, "Rather than viewing himself as bequeathing to the world a final solution to these issues, [he] saw himself as merely another participant . . . in an ongoing dialogue about some of the most urgent questions humanity faces in an age of science."[30]

Like Monod, Peacocke concerned himself throughout his career with questions on the meaning of life as evolved and evolving. Indeed, Peacocke believed that, in their lifelong journey of grappling with the dynamics and significance of evolution, he and Monod had a common origin: "I [have] suggested that Monod and I were at least fellow-voyagers setting out from the same home port of the scientific perspective on the world."[31] However, by bringing theological interpretations to evolution, Peacocke understood himself to be aiming for a very different destination than Monod:

> The course I have steered approaches a very different land-fall from that of Monod. I am not pretending that the journey by the route I have indicated will be any less stormy, indeed some nights may be darker, but, if we had time *to travel this route further*, I would suggest that a gleam of light could be discerned on the horizon, perhaps even that "day-spring from on high" which was promised us.[32]

Monod was a careful and daring scientific thinker who highlighted the function of chance in biological being. As a scientist, Peacocke responded to Monod by emphasizing the role of necessity alongside of chance in all evolutionary phenomena, including cancers. As a theologian, Peacocke added to his scientific observations on both random occurrences and law-like regularities his own belief that God was at work in them, but in a way that did not add anything observable to that work.

Next, we consider another—and a highly unusual—evolutionary thinker, Charles Sanders Peirce (1839–1914). While Peirce did not reflect on the evolution of cancer, he also died from the disease. We shall see how Peirce offers important insights into the possibilities and problems of

29. Peacocke, *All That Is*, 25.

30. Clayton, "Introduction," xv.

31. Peacocke, "Chance, Potentiality and God," 23.

32. Ibid.

understanding love—both divine and human—in a world of cancer chance and necessity.

Love and the Taming of Chance:
Charles Sander Peirce

It is hard to summarize the life of Peirce because Peirce led many lives. The son of a Harvard professor of mathematics, and himself a graduate of the college, he was, through an extended period of his early years, a coastal surveyor, and for a short period of time a professor of philosophy at Johns Hopkins University. After a forced and ignominious departure from Hopkins at the age of forty-four, Peirce remained mostly unemployed and became impoverished, even as William James periodically secured him short editing and essay-writing assignments. His career contained more twists and turns, but throughout its flux, there were two constants: one was his theorizing about and practicing science. The other was employing that science to hypothesize on the first principles (or metaphysics) of the world: "My philosophy may be described as the attempt of a physicist to make such conjecture as to the constitution of the universe as the methods of science may permit, with the aid of all that has been done by previous philosophers."[33]

Among Peirce's abiding scientific/philosophical efforts was to determine the first principles of evolutionary processes during an era when "agnosticism was then riding its high horse and was frowning superbly upon all metaphysics."[34] A poetic paraphrase of Peirce's own descriptions of meetings by a "Metaphysical Club" in the late 1800s reflects how this community of inquiry strove to make meaning of evolution: "A knot of us . . . gathered to discuss metaphysical/questions force law fate Darwin."[35] The labors of this conversational ensemble helped birth American pragmatism—a movement that proposed to a scientific age focused on facts and evidence that thoughts and ideas were not inconsequential, but had their own empirical effects and practical bearings. As pragmatism developed, its proponents continued to express this central conviction in a variety of ways, and, later in his life, Peirce did so this way: "It is a perfectly intelligible opinion that ideas. . . have a power of finding or creating their vehicles [in

33. Peirce, *Collected Papers*, 1.7.
34. Ibid., 5.12.
35. Related by Howe, *Pierce-Arrow*, 66.

the minds of humans], and having found them, of conferring upon them the ability to transform the face of the earth."[36]

Of course, some of these transformations are for the better, and others are not; for example, certain ideas may lead people to harm others, while other ideas may influence them to help others. But in these cases and in many others, ideas do have power to create new facts in the world. In particular, Peirce proposed as a testable hypothesis that the principle of love could affect the course of evolution. And he suggested that humanity had a role in bringing about this change for a more harmonious—and, ultimately, more loving—universe.

Peirce was a philosopher open to a mix of religious and scientific thought, and nowhere was this availability more apparent than in his analysis of evolution. He parsed out three dynamisms at work in not only within life, but throughout the cosmos.

> Three modes of evolution have thus been brought before us: evolution by fortuitous variation, evolution by mechanical necessity, and evolution by creative love. . . . The . . . propositions that absolute chance, mechanical necessity, and the law of love are severally operative in the cosmos may receive the names of *tychism*, *anancism*, and *agapism*.[37]

Having observed and recorded regularities in his coastal surveys, Peirce thought it incontrovertible that a dynamism best described as "necessity" directs the flow of events throughout the world. Yet, while he appreciated how the concept of necessity helps frame many mechanics of nature, Peirce found it inadequate to explain the innumerable free-flowing currents also coursing throughout creation. To account for this persistent "blooming and buzzing confusion,"[38] as William James described it, Peirce turned to chance as an enduring force: "Everywhere the main fact is growth and increasing complexity . . . . There is probably in nature some agency by which the complexity and diversity of things can be increased. . . . The theory of chance merely consists in supposing this diversification does not antedate all time."[39] Peirce believed creation itself reveled in the force of chance, because chance allowed creation to continue to create—to birth new, complicated and, often, higher forms of being into the world.

36. Peirce, *Collected Papers*, 1.220.
37. Ibid., 6.302.
38. James, *The Principles of Psychology*, 462.
39. Peirce, *Collected Papers*, 1.65.

While new being emerges from chance, so, too, does chaos. As a philosopher with strong moral sensibilities, Peirce therefore wondered if all this evolutionary chance and necessity might have some endpoint or purpose. As a scientist addressing an era also struggling with the social implications of differing and frequently competing evolutionary theories, Peirce claimed he could discern in the world a third force, that of love, at work through chance and necessity and directing it toward a harmonious state of being. To support this claim, Peirce referenced findings by physicists that many initially chaotic conditions such as gaseous states eventually do settle down. He also pondered the statistical properties of the law of large numbers (the same we noted in coin tossing and gambling) for indications that the oddities brought on by chance might eventually even out. To be sure, because chance occurrences are inevitable, creation will always have instabilities; otherwise, there could be no new being. But Peirce conjectured that, over time, chance might gradually be tamed and its rough places made so plain that they would become negligible.[40]

Peirce used many strategies to schematize how love might bring about such a positive transformation of the natural order. Among the talents Pierce possessed was the mathematical thinking his father had mastered, and so he employed the mathematical figure of asymptote to exhibit his hypothesis that the harmonious practical bearings of love might, over time, lessen the effects of chance: when a line and curve are asymptotic, the distance between them gradually approaches, though does not reach, zero as they extend themselves toward infinity (see Figure 5).

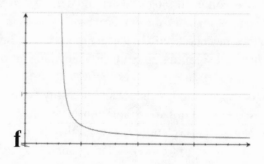

Figure 5: Asymptote

Peirce proposed that, similarly, love may gradually tame chance, so that chance will come infinitesimally close to meeting up with love.

40. Hacking, *The Taming of Chance*, 315.

Prima facie, Peirce's notion about "Evolutionary Love" may seem to be fanciful at best—an exotic religion and science cocktail whose ingredients really do not blend well. Some scholars contend that, by itself his science of evolution is an incoherent mix of Darwinian and anti-Darwinian elements. We, ourselves, share the particular concern that Peirce's thoughts on the power of love to make the world more peaceful contain components of a somewhat naïve late–nineteenth-century optimism that the world will, sooner or later, turn out to be a better place.

In the end, however, something not only attractive but also plausible persists in Peirce's notion that love is drawing the world toward better ends—for that idea, in true pragmatic fashion, may have the practical effect of leading persons to act lovingly toward one another and the world. Peirce himself understood it that way: that it was not only the idea of gospel love that could transform the world, but also the conduct of those who acted in sympathy with that idea. "Under this conception, the ideal of conduct is to execute our little function in the operation of the creation by giving a hand toward rendering the world more reasonable whenever, as the slang is, it is 'up to us: to do so.'"[41]

Peirce's proposal about agape was a bold one: under its sway, humanity might tame chance for the purpose of greater harmony and less suffering. And his notion may appear less a flight of fancy if we ground it in the more general pragmatic principle that ideas may have great power, sometimes for ill and hopefully for good.

Still, while bold and hopeful, our question is this: what might this theory about love working through chance and necessity, in fact, mean for cancer? That is, what might be the practical bearings of Peirce's evolutionary love for a theology of cancer? On the face of it, Peirce's theory of evolutionary love may not seem to signify much of anything for our particular purposes. That is so because, in its destructive authority over other cells, the evolution of cancer through chance and necessity does not seem to be tending toward any kind of harmonious conclusion. As cancers develop and continue along their evolutionary course, the line of love that might bring about a diminution of cancer suffering appears to remain remote from the line of cancerous developments and their suffering.

Which leads us to the primary question of our inquiry: what is love and where is God amidst the chance and necessity of cancers?

41. Peirce, *Collected Papers*, 1.615.

Chance, Necessity, Love . . . and Cancer

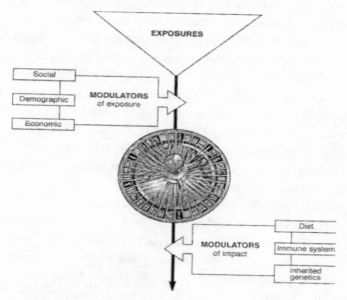

MUTATION SET

Inherited → IIIIIIIIIIIIIIIIIIIIIIIIIIIIIIIIIIIIIIII → FULL HOUSE,
CLONAL ESCAPE

Mutation   TIME

Figure 1: A prescription for composite risk of cancer (reproduced
permission from Mel Greaves, *Cancer: The Evolutionary Legacy*.
Oxford: Oxford University Press, 2001, Figure 23.1, 214).

In the introduction to our inquiry into an evolutionary theology of cancer,
we considered the figure above and asked wherein God and love might be
discerned. Having surveyed several thinkers on chance, necessity, and love,
we return to the diagram with which we began and ask what perspectives
we now might bring to it.

First, we meditate on this diagram from the worldview offered us by
Monod. Looked at this way, God is nowhere apparent amidst the events
depicted therein. Instead, if we zoom in and look closely at each of these
many elements, we see only the workings out of chance. First it is never
necessary that, at any given instant, the "Exposures" (brought on by both
intra- and extra-cellular events), noted at the top of the chart, will occur.

Next, not only is the occurrence of particular "Modulators of Exposure" always a matter of chance, but so is the mediation of their effects (as depicted in central image of the roulette wheel) on various populations. It is always by chance that a single genetically mutated cell (as pictured in the bottom of the chart) might emerge within an individual, and, furthermore, whether that cell will succeed in acquiring the requisite genetic mutations ("full house") to become a true cancer is always a bet. "Chance alone is at the source of every innovation, of every creation in the realm of life" (Monod), or, at least from this perspective, the source of the innovative creations of and by cancers. And from the perspective of Greaves, chance may also turn up as the "joker in the pack" that increases the likelihood of the "full house of clonal escape."[42]

From the scientific perspective of Peacocke (and all the others who share his understanding of the role of "necessity" in evolutionary phenomena), we see not only all the above, but also much more. That is, while we perceive the hinges of chance events upon which the development of cancers turn, we also discern various law-like regularities that govern their effects. Thus, both the arrows and the very flow of the chart portray directionalities that cannot be reversed. Rather, these laws "canalize" the course of chance occurrences toward the development of cancers.

To be sure, as cancers progress, chance remains in force so that not all potential cancers will have a hit at the roulette wheel nor will each be dealt the requisite cards for a full house. Thus, if any of the particular elements in this graph are altered by chance, the flow may be disrupted. On the other hand, if we look less at these individual elements, and, zooming out, focus on the big picture of their interconnectedness whenever cancers do happen to occur, we are faced with what Greaves himself saw in this graph: the statistical certainty that, in fact, cancers will occur somewhere, sometime, and that they will likely develop more among certain persons rather than others.[43]

From Peacocke's theological perspective, is God apparent in the chance and in the necessity depicted here? Yes and no. Peacocke believed that God was also at work in the chance and necessity of cancers, but that the particulars of these divine labors were not discernible and could not be depicted. Furthermore, he believed that God is in no way divorced from the

42. Greaves, *Cancer*, 27.

43. "Cancer then becomes a statistical inevitability in nature—a matter of chance and necessity, to quote Jacques Monod's memorable phrase, applied to evolution"; ibid., 52.

pain and suffering of the world brought on by these evolutionary dynamics: "God suffers with creation and in the creative process—that is, God *is* Love."[44] From this perspective, all that is in the world is the body of Christ, including all that is pictured in Greaves's graphic about cancer's destructive progression.

And from the perspective of Peirce, we finally ask: do we see love leading the evolutionary chance and necessity of cancer toward a more harmonious and loving end? As noted, apparently not, for in the sovereignty of cancer cells over cells for their own deadly purposes, love does not appear to be the be-all and end-all of cancers. Accordingly, we might conclude that, even though Peirce labored hard to demonstrate that divine love was pulling along all things in this world toward a good conclusion, nowhere is such love apparent in this cancerous progression.

However, the above is not our conclusion based on Peirce's perspective. Rather, it is this:

> Our loving efforts, enacted in sympathy with God's love for the world and in empathy for the evolutionary nature of the world, may testify to divine love amidst the evolutionary chance and necessity of cancers. First, by using our scientific understanding of cancer in the world, we may bring about transformations in the world of cancers. Furthermore, we may bring theological interpretations to the chance and necessity of cancers that witness to the love of God in, with, and under their evolutionary development.

This constitutes our thesis of an evolutionary theology of cancer. We develop that thesis in the following sections.

Chance, Necessity, Love: An Evolutionary Theology of Cancer

We may divide the thesis above into two separate but related proposals:

> (1) Through their research, scientific "communities of inquiry" strive to understand and increasingly succeed at understanding the evolutionary nature of cancers. The efforts of these communities, carried out by persons both of faith and of no faith, witness to the love of God present in, with, and under, the evolution of cancers. (2) Through religious reflection on the chance and necessity of the disease of cancer, we have the ability to construct

44. Peacocke, "God's Action in the Real World," 474.

meaning about that evolutionary phenomenon. These theological constructions may reveal and make real God's love for this world with cancers in it.

We begin with the first proposal: that God may be understood to be at work through human efforts of scientific inquiry.

Chance, Necessity, and Divine Love in the Science of Cancer

In the first section of our evolutionary theology of cancer, we provided a narrative of cancer as a disease of cells and of genes that has distinctive evolutionary hallmarks—and then, in a practical theological manner, we have subsequently employed that narrative as the "situation" for which our evolutionary theology has offered faithful understandings and wise responses. While the narrative about cancer that we have created for this book and then handed on to you, the reader, is our own, it is not ours alone. First, it derives from what has been handed on to us through the research of numerous past and present cancer scientists. Second, our narrative is part of the larger and productive family of contemporary retellings of this research that we have referenced—e.g, that of Greaves, Bishop, and Mukherjee.

The link, then, between our unique rendition of basic cancer science and these others, past and present, is that all are part of what Peirce described as a community of inquiry—those formal and informal networks whereby persons exchange and together test out ideas. That is why one reviewer of Mukherjee's biography of cancer notes a commonality between the way knowledge unfolded in his chronicle of cancer science and the emergence of ideas through the labors of Peirce's Metaphysical Club: both were birthed by communities of inquiry engaged in a collective striving to understand.[45]

The method by which cancer scientists have generated information for our narrative is their back and forth posing and testing of hypotheses to account for the way cancers come and go. This method of inquiry—formulating theories about the way cancers behave and then, through empirical trial and error, determining whether those theories appear to be true or false—is the means by which these communities, in the words of Monod, "try to understand" the origin and development of cancers. In doing so,

45. "'The Emperor of All Maladies' and Louis Menand."

none of these proposals have included God as an element or cause to account for the nature of cancers.

To explain why they have not, we turn to the famous story of the astronomer and mathematician, Pierre-Simon Laplace (1749–1827), who, when questioned by Napoleon Bonaparte why God was nowhere mentioned in his large tome on the order of the universe, replied, *Je n'avais pas besoin de cette hypothèse-là.* "I had no need of that hypothesis."[46] In trying to understand natural phenomena, the scientific community of inquiry does not employ religious signs or symbols to explain their origins and processes. Nor in our collaborative inquiry as a theologian and scientist have we employed God as a hypothesis to report findings from cancer science for an evolutionary theology of that disease.

Why have we included study of the world as if God were not given in it, or to it, or even for it in an evolutionary theology of cancer? We turn again to George Murphy's thoughts on kenosis for an understanding of how the love of God may be understood to be at work in, with, and under these particular scientific attempts to understand cancer: "a scientific theory *should* be 'a-theistic' in the precise sense that the concept of God does not appear as an element of the theory itself."[47] The religious reason for appreciating this a-religious perspective on nature may be explicated this way: the God of creation is a God who, "wills for something to exist that is not God."[48]

God's doing so permits a scientific enterprise that does not take God into account in order to study this creation:

> The ability to understand the world comes to fullest expression in science. . . . The very possibility of scientific understanding is grace. We might conceive of God acting [in the world] in accord with some higher rationality that cannot be grasped by creatures within the world. What is critical for the existence of scientific understanding is that God voluntarily limits divine action to be in accord with the rationality that God has conferred upon the world, so that creation can be understood as "though God were not a given."[49]

Out of love, God has created a world of chance and necessity about which some knowledge may be attained through the assumptions and procedures

46. De Morgan, ed., *A Budget of Paradoxes*, 2.
47. Murphy, *The Cosmos in the Light of the Cross*, 116.
48. Ibid., 84.
49. Ibid., 85.

of science. Thus, while considerations of nature as if God were not given might initially appear to be at cross-purposes with a Christian understanding of creation, viewed from the perspective of a theology of the cross, we may see that doing so may assist us in understanding the natural operations of the world.

We add the following for an evolutionary theology of cancer: graced by God's love, we are called to consider the nature of cancer through scientific study without the hypothesis of God. Furthermore, by the grace of God, we may use such scientific study of cancer—atheistic in its methodology—to further God's purposes for this world. A review of some key points of what we have learned about basic cancer science will illustrate how this is so.

Throughout our inquiry into the nature of cancer, we have highlighted how it is not a simple disease. To be sure, cancer may be easily described as a disease of cells—of the very constitutive elements of our bodies and being. Yet, cancer is not simply the disordered inner workings of any one or many cancerous cells, but the disorder that results from the complicated network of relationships that those cells establish with normal cells.[50] We also have portrayed cancer, on the one hand, as a disease of genes within cells, and it is most certainly that. On the other hand, as cancers progress with reference to the genetic library, the genome itself is often transformed into a bewildering chaos. And, while this disease of cells and genes does unfold through space and over time according to some very identifiable evolutionary hallmarks, the occurrence and timing of these typical features appear in novel ways in every individual case of cancer—and they do so precisely because every event of biological evolution is a unique phenomenon. So, to be sure, common features do exist among cancers, but, with their intrinsic variability, cancers find ever new ways to develop.[51] Indeed, as we have noted, it is quite possible that cancer is the most complex disease that exists.

Nevertheless, we have demonstrated that along with their complexity, cancers have contours that may be grasped, i.e., "comprehended." That is, we now do have a clear and distinct idea of what cancers are, and our understanding of cancers is as sure and certain as it gets: cancers are cells that go their own way according to evolutionary dynamisms of chance

---

50. In the words of D. W. Smithers, "Cancer is no more a disease of cells than a traffic jam is a disease of cars. A lifetime's study of the internal combustion engine will not explain it"; Smithers, "Cancer an Attack," 493.

51. See again Kitano, "Cancer as a Robust System."

and necessity. Running throughout the chaos of this disease of cells and genes, with its telltale hallmarks, are these very principles of evolutionary development that, themselves, are comprehensible and provide us a means of wrapping our understanding around the phenomenon of cancers. Furthermore, we can now not only outline the fundamental features of cancers, but we can also fill in details of those features more precisely. Because of our efforts, cancer is, in Bishop's language, less a closed "black box" and more an open one so that we may now better determine the genetic events required to initiate it and then to move it along.

To be sure, the course of our increasingly precise knowledge of cancer has not been straight and smooth, but rather long and winding. That progress has been uneven because our knowledge of this evolutionary disease has itself been evolving through chance discoveries and subsequent integration of those findings. And as Peirce noted, all scientific efforts miss the mark of a final truth even as their conclusions may increasingly cluster around the bull's eye of such a truth. Accordingly, we may never arrive at a complete understanding of cancers, nor may we ever arrive at a full understanding of their origins and development that would enable us to prevent or cure all of them.

However, we are progressing closer to better understandings of cancers that may enable us to better cope with them. Accordingly, Peirce's words about all scientific inquiry apply to cancer research: "Despair is insanity. True, there may be facts that will never get explained but . . . we must be guided by the rule of hope."[52] Our increasingly precise understandings of the inner workings of cancers are themselves the practical bearings of inquiry guided by hope.

Our improved scientific understanding of both the contours and inner features of cancers has born another particularly good fruit: our increased ability to intervene as the disease develops. To the degree that we understand cancers to be phenomena of evolution, to that degree we are thereby enabled to treat and, in some cases, to cure those with it. That is, the more we understand how cancers progress according to evolutionary principles, the better we are to able adapt to them and, in some cases, to create ways to overcome them.

To be sure, evolution is the very dynamism that predicts that cancers will always develop somewhere, sometime. But with our understanding of the ways in which cancers are evolutionary events, we may now better

52. Peirce, *Collected Papers*, 1.405.

predict their ways and, through various interventions, outflank their development. Throughout our study, we have offered brief examples of how we may do so and, in a subsequent chapter, we will elaborate on how we may redirect the flow of cancerous chance and necessity.

If we revisit Greaves's graph and ask where love might be discerned amidst the evolutionary development depicted therein, we may now offer several answers. First, we may confess God's love to be at work in our very ability to understand the dynamics of chance and necessity involved in the progression of cancers sketched out in such graphs. Love may also be found in our ability derived from this science to intervene at many points along the figure to control some exposures that may initiate cancers (e.g. tobacco) and to affect modulators of their exposure and impact. That is, our comprehension of cancers may enable us to transform their evolutionary processes, and, thereby, become a way that God may work in, with, and under those processes to produce a world with less pain and suffering.

While the findings of cancer science may not be able to reveal the workings of God in nature, they may be means by which we can further God's purposes for nature. Accordingly we may confess that all members of the cancer science "community of inquiry"—including those who profess belief in a God and those who do not—may be doing the work of the Lord whenever they research cancers as if there were no God. For example, we can understand the practical bearings of Monod's thought in each and every one of the previously cataloged articles that build on his work as instruments by which divine love may be operative in a world of chance and necessity. With the eyes of faith, we may review that long list of previously cited research derived from Monod's atheistic speculations on chance and necessity as godly products by which we have been enabled to cut into the evolutionary phenomenon of cancer. To the degree that similar attempts by other researchers bring about better understandings of the world that may lead to better treatment for those with the disease, such attempts may be received as the work of God in the world.

How does this theology of divine love at work in, with, and under our scientific understandings and efforts connect with those that we have already considered? Earlier we examined a theological position that God has created a world in which cancers are inevitable—a fact that we, in faith, may learn to accept and, even, to offer our consent. We also summarized another, somewhat different, theological perspective that we may hope that God intends to bring us some kind of deliverance from cancers. We find our proposal that God works through science both to provide us with a comprehension of cancers and to bring about a world with less cancer, death, and suffering incorporates key elements of each of these positions. On the one hand, it takes into account that there may be no final removal of these sources of suffering because they are built into the structure of being. Accordingly, we are called to faithfully face the fact that the persistent presence of cancers in this world may be a part of divine intent.

On the other hand, the proposal that God may be at work through our scientific endeavors to reduce the pain and suffering shows an appreciation for the power of continuing creation. In the world of the finite—and in God's time stretched out infinitely before us—we may be guided by the hope that the asymptotic distinction between the reality of cancers and the power of divine/human love may so diminish that cancerous suffering would still obtain, but, being an infinitesimal distinction, might no longer be perceivable or be experienced.

In sum, the science of cancer may offer us tools to respond wisely to a world with cancers by helping us to learn to accept what cannot be changed about them and also to hope to change what can be. Again, by wise responses, we mean in the biblical sense those that enable us to "*to cope* with reality, be it favorable or threatening."[53] And, again, we conceive of these responses as those whose practical bearings provide us tools "of . . . reshaping as much of the environment as is within our power in order to destroy the factors in the universe that work against our well-being and even our very survival."[54]

Now, considering our second proposal, we shall examine more closely faithful understandings of the world as if God were not given amidst the chance and necessity of cancer. In doing so, we shall see how these theological proposals support not only scientific endeavors without consideration of God amidst the chance and necessity of cancer but also endeavors to make religious meaning of this evolutionary process.

God's Love in, with, and under the Chance and Necessity of Cancer

We have noted that George Murphy offers a religious appreciation of the world that does not include God as an explanatory factor for scientific

53. Crenshaw, *Old Testament Wisdom*, 230.
54. Smith, *The Spirit of American Philosophy*, 21.

inquiry into its operations. Because he understands God in Christ to have given of God's self through the act of creation, Murphy believes that creation itself may be interpreted through scientific inquiry, "though God were not given (*etsi deus non daretur*)" or, in the related concept, "as if God were not given (*acsi deus non daretur*)."[55] Coined by the Dutch jurist and natural philosopher Hugo Grotius (1583–1645), these concepts have gained theological currency from their use by Dietrich Bonhoeffer to dismiss a God of the gaps, and by Eberhard Jüngel to argue for the worldly non-necessity of God. In this section, we expand the religious rationale for not needing God to explain the operations of the world with cancer in it, and, consequently, for also needing a host of religious symbols through which God offers meaning for that world.

We connect our own understanding of both God's hiddenness in the world and the need for religious meanings of God's love in the midst of that hiddenness with one we noted earlier: Martin Luther's typology of theologies of glory and theologies of the cross. In his 1518 treatise, "The Heidelberg Disputation," Luther described theologies of glory as efforts to detail the ways in which God is at work in the world for the good of the world. Contra such theologies, Luther contended that God's ways in the world are matters about which we, by faith, may have only have clues or indicators. Believing that God both reveals Godself from creation and also remains hidden under creation, he derided all attempts to demonstrate God's glory in creation as inevitably frustrating and foolish.

Not only does God hide God's self from the world, but God also puts on a mask in God's revelation to and relationship with it—and God's doing so is the subject matter of theologies of the cross that consider Christ's improbable manner of dying on an instrument of execution. Centuries later, Hegel offered his own summary of this theology's construal of God's relationship with the cosmos:

> "God himself is dead," it says in a Lutheran [Good Friday] hymn, expressing an awareness that the human, the finite, the fragile, the weak, the negative are themselves a moment of the divine, that they are within God's very self, that finitude, negativity, otherness are not outside of God and do not . . . hinder unity with God.[56]

---

55. Murphy, *The Cosmos in Light of the Cross*, 5. Murphy also employs throughout his book Thomas Torrance's preferred phrase, *acsi deus non daretur*, "as if God were not given."

56. Hegel, *Lectures*, 326.

Luther himself never quite said that God died on a cross but did pinpoint God's presence there as well as the transcendence of God in confounding human understanding in that hidden revelation.

Another source for appreciating approaches to the world as if God were not given is available in letters Dietrich Bonhoeffer wrote before his execution by the Nazis: "The God who lets us live in the world without the working hypothesis of God is the God before whom we stand continually. Before God and with God we live without God."[57] Drawing on Grotius, Bonhoeffer argued that homo sapiens need not morph into homo religiosis in order to know the world, nor need the world itself be "religiocified" in order to be understood.

Of course, discourse about God's apparent absence from or actual death in the cosmos could be expressions of and inducements toward varieties of atheistic experience. The contention by Ludwig Feuerbach (1804–1872) that Luther's essence of faith was essentially faith in human ideals and possibilities before the limits of the world was a bit of both. However, there are faithful ways of appropriating this language, as indicated in the very title of the book, *God as the Mystery of the World: On the Foundation of the Theology of the Crucified One in the Dispute between Theism and Atheism*, by Eberhard Jüngel. Rather than dismissing modern atheism, Jüngel takes it and runs with it in order to give the dignity due to both the God and the world. That is, Jüngel concurs with atheists like Feuerbach and Nietzsche that God is not necessary for world to be what it is. Rather, he argues that God is "more than necessary" for the world since God is the very meaning and mystery of the world.[58]

Rather than searching for the meaning of God in the world through analysis of its contingencies and laws, we may search instead for the meaning of the world with these features within the love of the crucified God for creation. "Jüngel's point is not that God lacks excellence [by not being necessary to explain the operations of the world], but rather we must learn what is truly good and excellent in the world by looking at God."[59] We, ourselves, concur with Jüngel's proposition that God is hiddenly present in the suffering brought on by cancers as well as in indicators of God's purpose to deliver us from its suffering.

57. Bonhoeffer, *Letters and Papers*, 360.
58. Jüngel, *God as the Mystery of the World*, 33.
59. Dehart, *Beyond the Necessary*, 159.

While our good works in and for the world are ways that God does God's work, God still remains hidden under and concealed (or "masked") by our own efforts on God's behalf. "What else is all our work to God, whether in the fields, in the garden, in the city, in the house, in war, or in government, but just such a child's performance, by which He wants to give His gifts in the fields, at home and everywhere else? These are the masks of God, behind which He wants to remain concealed and do all things."[60]

As a way in which love may show itself within and, thereby, direct the course of the world toward a better outcome, Peirce had proposed that humanity has a "function in creation by giving a hand." Luther similarly claims that our good works may be means by which God's good will for creation is realized in it. "We have the saying: 'God gives every good thing, but not just by waiving a wand.' God gives all good gifts; but you must lend a hand and take the bull by the horns, that is you must work and thus give God good cause and a mask."[61] Luther described medical knowledge as one means of God's putting on a human disguise to go about God's business—and it is no stretch of the fundamentals of his theology to include, as Murphy has, scientific inquiry as a process that both reveals and masks God's good work for the world that God loves.

In sum: the various perspectives noted above converge in discerning that, while there is no need for the "working hypothesis of God" to explain natural operations of the world, God is at work in them. Just as God reveals God's self on a cross, a place where we might expect God not to wind up, so God is at work both through the purposeless processes of natural evolution and also through scientific efforts to study these processes as if God were not present in them. And, just as God's working out of God's purposes on a cross is not clearly apparent, equally imperceptible are God's good purposes for the world through nature.

Peacocke describes how we may utilize scientific explanations of nature in which God's work is not apparent in order to further God's work for the world:

> In the history of Israel, God was always raising up apparent scourges, such as Cyrus, that were in reality blessings in disguise leading his people through the trauma that would alone enable them to apprehend new truths. So it is with evolutionary biology

60. Luther, *Luther's Works* 14:114–5.
61. Ibid.

which . . . for Christian theology under the disguise of a foe, did
the work of a friend.[62]

The good news for Peacocke, and for us, is that events such as cancer that
appear to be purposeless and even Godless, through accounts of evolution
offered by Monod and others with his worldview, are not outside the providence of God.

While this theology of God's cruciform love for the world in, with, and
under its evolutionary processes proclaims that God's ways in the world are
not apparent, through this very proclamation it also offers us narratives and
symbols of God's concern for the world. In doing so, this theology of God's
love resonates with the faithful understandings and wise responses found
in other theologies that we have previously considered. The love of God is
the leitmotif of those theologies that call on us to wisely respond by letting
go and letting be in this world in response to God's own *Gelassenheit* in
creating a world that is something other than God's self. And it is the love of
God for creation that motivates those theologies that hope for a redeemed
creation—and also hope that, as part of that redemption, God will bring a
purpose to the world that may not now be found in it.[63] Both these theological positions offer stories and symbols that communicate ways in which
God loves the world of evolutionary chance and necessity. And they express
a common faith in the God whose work in creation is not apparent except
to faith, and has no purpose in God's self except whose ultimate concern is
to love what God has created.

This love of God for creation is communicated through theologies
that employ symbols about and narratives of God's love. Similarly, throughout all the theologizing on the evolutionary phenomenon of cancer that
we have reviewed, religious symbols and narratives have been brought to
bear on the chance and necessity of cancer. By these efforts, theologians are
"lending God a hand," and thereby demonstrating another way in which
divine love may show itself amidst this chance and necessity. That is this:
through the symbols and stories that theologians deploy about the chance
and necessity of cancer, they may help to reveal the love of God in a world
with cancers in it. While theological study may not afford insight keener
than scientific inquiry into the operations of nature, it is a means by which

62. Peacocke, *Evolution*, 49.

63. "We . . . avoid locating purpose or direction or even value *within nature; yet, we
. . . affirm a divine* purpose *for nature*"; Peters and Hewlett, *Evolution from Creation to
New Creation*, 28.

we may offer faithful understandings into the evolutionary nature of God's world in which cancers occur.

How might symbols, both those that are explicitly religious and those that are not, bring purpose to a world of chance and necessity? We may consider how symbols employ these evolutionary forces of chance and necessity to communicate meaning and purpose by considering the example of Holy Communion. By chance, all the elements required—including bread, wine, a gathering of persons—may come together so that the practice might take place. Furthermore, in any occurrence of such communion, law-like regularities predict who will be present and who will not be, and, also, laws of nature are at work in the physical processes of the pouring of wine for drinking and in the transmission of sound waves by which words of institution are heard. But to understand the meaning and significance of this religious practice, one must consider not only such random occurrences and law-like regularities but also the transforming word of God as operative in, with, and under them.

For sure, not all efforts at meaning making, both of the religious sort and other kinds, may be understood to be the work of the Lord, since, as we have noted, even those that are theologically informed may lead some people to do ungodly things. Furthermore, all divine symbols may be used idolatrously—e.g., consecrated elements of Holy Communion may be desecrated and quests for the Holy Grail may be ideal but also may bring real harm to others. So, while they are integral to the transformation and reformation of life, all symbols and practices may become deformed and thereby become deadly for human spirit and for human life.

Our consideration of this second proposal whereby divine love may be discerned amidst the evolutionary phenomenon of cancer can be summarized this way: we are able to communicate God's love for a world of cancers by handing over revelations that have been handed down to us through various symbols of God at work through the chance and necessity of that disease. We may confess that, out of love, God has created a world in which cancers are inevitable because God's world is full of creative chance and ordering regularities. And we may proclaim that, also out of love, God has created a world in which we see indicators and possibilities for deliverance from sufferings that come from cancers. From the perspective afforded us by a theology of the cross, we may appreciate, to paraphrase Hegel, how all things human, finite, fragile, weak, and negative generated by the evolutionary phenomenon of cancer are themselves within God's very self and do not hinder unity with God. On the other hand, we may employ a cross-wise hermeneutic of suspicion that the highest ideals about and best practices related to cancer may fail to communicate the love of God because such ideals may be idolatrous and even best practices may take on bad forms.

Conclusion

In this chapter, we first reviewed the ways in which three thinkers grappled with the evolutionary principles of chance and necessity. We then considered the implications of their having done so for a theology of God's love in a world of cancerous chance and necessity. Doing so enabled us next to propose a thesis for an evolutionary theology whereby we may understand the love of God in a world with cancers to be at work in two ways: (1) scientific endeavors that help us to comprehend and sometimes to cut into their evolutionary development, and (2) symbols and stories of the love of God amidst their chance and necessity. In the conclusion that follows, we first shall employ this evolutionary theology of cancer to give examples of how the love of God may be present in these ways. And then we shall exhort others to give similar testimony.

Conclusion

F ollowing our study of cancer's chance and necessity in the earlier chapters of our book, we examined theologies of acceptance and of hope as two faithful and wise responses to its evolution—and, then, proposed two ways that divine and human love may be present amidst its chance and necessity. Now we will offer examples of these ways of (1) making theological meaning about the disease through symbols and stories and (2) employing science of cancer's evolutionary processes to outflank its development. Having offered these illustrations, we will note some of the bearings on pastoral care of attending to the evolutionary dimensions of cancer. Then we will conclude with recommendations for further theological study that would testify to the love of God in a world with cancers—and that, in doing so, bring love to that world.

The Love of God in Making Theological Meaning about Cancer

Enfolded in Love: Acceptance and Arthur Peacocke

As he was dying from cancer, Arthur Peacocke was surrounded by a community of scholars who examined his lifelong proposal that the love of God is at work in "all that is" in the world.[1] Peacocke appreciated a particular

1. Clayton, "Introduction."

effect of this attention. "It was only during this time that the enormity of what I had to face up to gradually dawned on me and this catalysed me to finishing off 'An Essay in Interpretation' concerned with a more naturalistic understanding of the Christian faith."[2] Peacocke's encounter with cancer precipitated not only his closing remarks on theology and science, but also an account of his own faith amidst the turbulence of evolutionary chance and necessity: "A few weeks before his death, Peacocke composed and circulated a final statement entitled "Nunc Dimittis," the Latin translation of the opening of Simeon's canticle in Luke 2:29–35: 'Lord, now lettest thou thy servant depart in peace, according to thy word: For mine eyes have seen thy salvation, which thou hast prepared before the face of all people.'"[3]

In his earlier meditations on Monod, Peacocke had predicted that he himself might meet up with existential struggles and storms along his life journey. As evident in our following summary of and commentary on this final testimony, Peacocke did have such encounters—as well as experiencing his anticipated vision of the "day-spring from on high."

> Up until July 2004 I was blessed with a long, healthy and fruitful life. In July 2004, in my eightieth year I was diagnosed not only with prostate cancer, but having it in an advanced form. This was an enormous shock to myself and my wife. . . . By [2005], I was taking an enormous range of pills, bouts of nausea were becoming frequent, and it was becoming less and less possible to envisage a normal life of any kind. I was trying to be stoic and trying not to inveigh against God for what was clearly going to be my fate—a fate I had not really envisaged or imagined.[4]

After a career replete with productivity and well-being, Peacocke received his diagnosis of an "advanced" (in his case, fatal) cancer as a heavy blow. In response both to learning that he had this disease and to experiencing consequent suffering, he strove to be "stoic"—a term that might mean many things but, in Peacocke's case, seems to signify simply that he was trying to control himself. What might Peacocke have been trying to contain within? He shared that he was attempting not to "inveigh against God"—and, perhaps despite himself, confessed thereby that he was tempted to do so. In

2. Peacocke, *All That Is*, 191.
3. Clayton, "Introduction," 3.
4. Peacocke, *All That Is*, 191.

using the word *inveigh*, Peacocke informs us that, despite his faith in God, he was drawn to protest vehemently against God.

What troubled Peacocke was the impending "fate" of his cancer that he had not predicted. Twice, he uses this term that connotes to all such as himself who are familiar with Monod the purported lack of purpose for life given the capriciousness of the world. Peacocke's chance meeting with what he had not "envisaged or imagined" impels him to pray for something more:

> Over the years I have given much thought and spilt much ink on the nature of God and God's interaction with people. Not surprisingly the subtler nuances of my deliberations have fallen away before the absolute conviction that God is love and eternally so. This remains the foundation of my prayers and thoughts for "underneath are the everlasting arms." This is not always easily experienced and it needs much concentrated meditation—the "black dog" of depression is sometimes difficult to expel.[5]

Here, Peacocke clearly articulates his foundational religious belief—that God is love in, with, and under all that is. At the same time, he also expresses his destabilizing existential despair in response to one thing that is—his prostate cancer. To describe the state of his soul, he employs Winston Churchill's menacing canine metaphor for depression. To maintain his conviction "that God is love and eternally so," he claims he must meditate on this belief. It appears, therefore, that as Peacocke's inducement to inveigh increased, so did his need to focus on his theological convictions. In this final account, the tension builds as Peacocke, having described his fundamental beliefs being torn at by temptations, next revealed that a major source of this existential struggle derived from the single subject with which he had wrestled throughout his career as a scientist and theologian:

> [My] concern[s] over the years has been the recurrence of what theologians call 'natural evil.' I have often attempted to illustrate the ambivalence of this concept, for example showing that what we call natural evil is a consequence of a divinely created law-like structure implementing the divine purpose to bring into existence intelligent persons. *The irony is that one of the examples I took was the role of mutations in DNA which are the basic source of evolution,*

5. Ibid., 192.

and so of the emergence of human beings—and also of cancer. This
[illness] is a new challenge to the integrity of my past thinking.[6]

It was Peacocke's fate to have begun his career studying the chance and
necessity of cancer, next to live well into a very ripe older age, but then to
abruptly experience both his work and life undone by the very subject of
his study—and in a manner that brought great physical discomfort and significant psychic insult. Throughout his life journey, Peacocke had advanced
the "naturalist" argument that sufferings brought on by "all that is" are not
evil because they are part of nature's fabric. Yet, when Peacocke was struck
down by the disease that came into being through the same processes that
brought him and all humanity into being, he was struck hard by that irony.
Again, that irony has been summarized elsewhere this way:

no changes in genes = no cancer;

no changes in genes = no evolution = no us.[7]

How might one make meaning of this—that human being cannot come to
be except through the very process that also can cause its being to cease?
How might one solve this problem?

Or is this a problem to be solved in the sense of its being a puzzle
that must or even can be pieced together? Or, rather, is it more among the
mysteries of human being that humans may come to accept? As he draws
near the end of his testimony, Peacocke offered the following answer. "I am
only enabled to meet this challenge by my root conviction that God is Love
as revealed supremely in the life, death and resurrection of Jesus the Christ.
However the fact remains that death for me is imminent and of this I have
no fear because of that belief."[8]

Peacocke concludes his testament by recollecting the famous story
of spiritual transformation recounted in Bede's history of the coming of
Christianity to the Kingdom of Northumbria in England (597). In his own
rendition of this testimony by a court advisor, Peacocke omitted Bede's concluding sentence that summarizes this Northumbrian's desire for insights
into the mystery of being: "Therefore, if this new teaching has brought any
more certain knowledge, it seems only right that we should follow it."[9] In

6. Ibid., 192–93; emphasis added.
7. Greaves, *Cancer*, 47.
8. Peacocke, *All That Is*, 193.
9. Bede, *Ecclesiastical History*, 130–1.

its stead, Peacocke shared his own account of having been enlightened: "I know that God is waiting for me to be enfolded in love."[10] This, then, is the knowledge toward which Peacocke oriented himself—or rather, the knowledge that appears to have oriented Peacocke toward his end: "Death comes to everyone and this is my time."[11] In the end, Peacocke did not receive the fact that his life and his death were rooted within the same evolutionary process to be a problem, but to be a mystery with which he could live as he was dying. In light of this understanding of divine love for him and all creation, he claimed that he could accept their connectedness—and testified that he could depart in peace.

Surrounded by a community and blessed with a tradition that informed his faith, Peacocke was able to confess the love of God that enabled him to both accept and consent to his cancer. Next, we consider the experience of love in community that has enabled Deanna Thompson to have hope amidst the chance and necessity of her cancer.

Love through Tangible Agents:
Hope and Deanna Thompson

In recounting her struggles after being diagnosed with stage four breast cancer and her hopes for "something more" than the threats it brought to her and her family, we noted earlier that Thompson confessed, "I don't pretend to have adequate answers" to how that something more might occur or even what it would be. Thompson does, however, have a clear sense of how both God's love has enabled her to have hope and various communities have mediated that love to her:

> But even as I admit ignorance on the details, I nevertheless take heart in the fact that the biblical images of life with God are consistently and inescapably communal. The Apostle Paul asserts that in hope *we* have been saved; he also insists that nothing can separate *us* from the love of God in Christ Jesus. At the heart of the vision of life beyond this one is the affirmation of continued connection, of life in community.[12]

10. Peacocke, *All That Is*, 193.
11. Ibid.
12. Thompson, *Hoping for More*, 146.

Earlier we noted that many theologians of hope intentionally work backward from their eschatological vision of a redeemed existence in the future in order to discern God's good purpose for creation as it is now. In a way, Thompson reverses the sequence of such theological thinking as she imagines what eternal life might be like by projecting onto it her current experiences with those who love her and those whom she loves. With this foretaste fresh in her soul, she anticipates a feast to come.

> My life-altering experiences of community since the diagnosis—from my graced relationships with my husband and daughters to my exponentially expanded notion of the church universal to the vision of the heavenly banquet in the form of a quilting bee—have convinced me that despite knowing little of the details about life with God beyond this one, I've been granted faith that it will look something like the banquets of grace to which I've already been treated.[13]

Throughout her memoir, Thompson reflects at length on the various loving communities that have been resources for her hoping. In this pointedly theological narrative, she also comments on and analyzes the beliefs that have sustained her in these communities:

> [T]hrough this cancer journey, I've also been awakened to a new—indeed, almost mystical—understanding of the church universal and of the healing effects it has had on the lives of me and my family. The body of Christ is no longer an abstract, intangible concept glossed over during the reciting of the creed. . . . The church universal has become a tangible agent of grace in my life, a gift of support that has accompanied me through the valley of the shadow of cancer.[14]

Here, Thompson claims she has realized that the consolation of God may be offered to those in need through the care of the church. This consolation in religious community itself is "embodied," and therefore, finds its way to her, not through that which is "abstract" or via some "intangible concept" but in the "tangible agen[cy]" of supportive persons.

In her elaboration of experiencing community care, Thompson reports novel ways in which the love of others has been handed on to her. "What's been particularly surprising to me is that the experience of the church universal has been mediated through what I'm calling *the virtual*

13. Ibid.
14. Ibid., 57.

body of Christ; that is, the body of Christ incarnated in, with, and through the power of Internet sites like Caring Bridge."[15]

Through her invocation of terms *in, with,* and *through,* Thompson connects with what her tradition teaches about the ways in which God appears in the world. Through her particular use of these prepositions, though, it is not God who shows up in an unexpected manner, but the church that connects with her via the unexpected medium of Internet technology. And using the language of this tradition, Thompson offers a perspective that re-envisions the concept of community and gives new meaning to "embodiment." "What I'm talking about is a new understanding of the church universal, a breathtakingly broad embodiment of Christ's hands and feet ministering amidst the sorrows and joys of our world. I'm talking about Christ made present to me and my family through the connections made possible by a website."[16]

Through this technological medium, Thompson also experiences community with other Christians with whom many other forms of communion, including Holy Communion, are now not possible. "This experience of the virtual body of Christ has also gifted me with a fresh appreciation of the necessarily ecumenical character of church catholicity. Prompted by my entries on the Caring Bridge site, many of my friends from the Roman Catholic tradition—the church that holds most tightly to this notion of universality—have embodied Christ to me in stunning ways."[17]

However, such new ways of being in communion with other Christians is not the end point of Thompson's experience of embodied love. The boundaries of community expand so that the body of Christ may incorporate those of other faiths:

> When it comes to the church universal, then, my understanding has been broken open to a new beyond—beyond what we Christians are able to imagine, beyond tidy categories of what counts as religious and what doesn't. Since the diagnosis, I've received a sage blessing from a Native American colleague, been prayed for in the synagogues of friends and colleagues, had Buddhist meditation sessions dedicated to me; and Jesus has even been asked a favor

15. Ibid.
16. Ibid.
17. Ibid., 58.

by a Jewish friend who took a gamble on my behalf. I don't know what else to call it but grace.[18]

There are many ways to interpret Thompson's description of these expanding boundaries, but one way that reveals the abiding and sustaining presence of love amidst her encounter with the chance and necessity of cancer is suggested by these words: "With God, all things are possible." Near the end of her memoir throughout which she has offered candid accounts of her anguish and suffering, Thompson reports that she and her family suddenly experienced the unexpected: a remission of her stage four breast cancer. Along with profound relief and gratitude at this news, Thompson reports that she also experiences "terror" at the thought of possibly becoming again as ill as she once had been. Given these conflicting emotions, she reports, "I try to trust that with God all things are possible."[19]

What, then, is hope given the chance occurrence of such good news and given a cancer that, while not necessarily deadly, sometimes certainly is? Hope seems to be something like the anticipation of or the waiting for that which seems just about impossible. Through her encounter with novel means of communication and new forms of community, Thompson experiences God's love as unbounded. Thompson's encounter with these many things is, when considered *in toto*, the "something more" that nourishes her hope in a God whose love is greater than not only death but also all other limits that she and others may encounter from cancer.

Taming Cancer Chance and Necessity through Scientific Understanding

In this section, we develop the second major thesis of the book: through their scientific research, various "communities of inquiry" strive to understand and, increasingly, succeed at understanding the evolutionary phenomenon of cancers. The efforts of these communities, whether they are constituted by persons of faith or by persons of no faith, are themselves part of the evolutionary work of God. Not all evolutionary phenomena are inevitable, and humans have the ability to cut into the flow and thereby alter the course of many of them. Accordingly, amidst the chance and necessity of cancer, our efforts may produce, and increasingly have produced, better

18. Ibid., 61–62.
19. Ibid., 129.

scientific understandings of and treatments for cancer—and, in doing so, affect the evolutionary progression of particular cancers. In fact, understanding the evolutionary nature of cancer has led to the development of new therapies that can cure the disease.

We have discussed how cancer is a disease of evolution—at the level of the DNA, the cells, the whole organism. This evolutionary nature of cancer itself also affects its response to therapy. One of the most difficult problems with cancer is that as it evolves in the body, it also evolves in response to therapy; treatments that worked early in the development of the cancer often do not work well later because of cancer evolution.

The earliest therapy used for tumors was surgery, and this is still an effective strategy for some tumors, although it is rarely used alone. The idea was to remove as much of the tumor as possible and then to anticipate that it would not grow back; unfortunately, many cancer cells invade the surrounding normal tissue and even if there is the appearance that the cancer has been removed, a few cells remain and the cancer regrows at or near the site of the original. The types of cancers that can be treated exclusively with surgery are usually those that are encapsulated with tissue or that have not spread into the normal tissue in any way.

Following surgery, one of the next therapies used for treatment of cancer was radiation, discovered in Wurzburg, Germany in 1895 by Roentgen, who identified X-rays as a means for being able to "see through" water-containing tissue and leave boney structures as dense material observable after exposure to X-rays. Years later, Marie Curie discovered radium and realized its power to kill cancer cells and its possible use in therapy. To this day, more than half of the cancers in the US are treated with radiation (albeit with much greater precision and sophistication than the radium ampules used by the Curies) and often with great success. Why has radiation been so successful in treating cancer? The beams from the radiation can be targeted directly to the cancer, avoiding much of the normal tissues in the body, so that the side effects are minimized.

A study of the development of cancer-killing drugs reveals that one of the first was methotrexate, which was used to kill an embryonic type of cancer called choriocarcinoma and the second was cyclophosphamide to treat a lymphoma. Both chemotherapeutic drugs are still in use today and effective in treatment of many types of cancer. Why do they work? These cancer drugs target cells that are rapidly dividing, and most cancer cells are affected because frequent (rapid) cell division is a hallmark of cancer.

The problem, of course, is that some normal cells in the body are also dividing (including stem cells, bone marrow, hair follicles, and others) and as a consequence, side effects of chemotherapy include damage to these dividing normal cells resulting in hair loss, anemia, immune dysfunction, and others.

In recent years there has been a strong emphasis on the development of targeted therapies to destroy cancers. This work has led to the identification of "driver" mutations and "passenger" mutations. Those driver mutations become the drivers of the evolution of the cancer, shaping how it will develop in the patient and what important features it will gain to make it thrive in that particular patient's environment. The recognition of this concept and the identification of specific driver mutations has given researchers critical points in the cancer evolution where they can design drugs to intervene and thwart the further development of the cancer. The recognition that cancer itself is an evolutionary process has been critical in the development of many modern therapies.

Targeted therapies have been developed that attempt to destroy some important target in the cancer cell that is not as vital for normal cells. The first targeted cancer therapy was directed against the estrogen receptor, which is expressed in estrogen-receptor-positive breast cancers. This drug, tamoxifen, attacked the cancer cells that were estrogen positive and prevented estrogen from regulating cancer cells and helping them to grow. Estrogen receptor dysregulation was later found to be a type of "driver" for genetic change leading to the development of breast cancer.

Another early targeted and successful therapy was developed for the treatment of chronic myelogenous leukemia (CML). CML is noteworthy because 95 percent of the patients with CML have a special change in the cellular chromosomes that give the cells a particular marker called the "Philadelphia chromosome" (so named because it was first identified in Philadelphia). This Philadelphia chromosome has pieces of two different chromosomes merged together, creating a unique structure not found in normal cells, making a unique protein that is the merger of two proteins not found in normal cells. This new protein became a unique target for a new chemotherapeutic drug developed in the laboratory to specifically treat CML; it now appears to be a driver mutation for induction of CML.

The drug called Gleevac (also called Imantinib) took about ten years from discovery of the Philadelphia chromosome to its development and has been remarkably effective in treatment of CML cases that have the

Philadelphia chromosome. This drug has also been shown to be effective against several other types of tumors with changes in proteins similar to those found in cancers carrying the Philadelphia chromosome. Gleevac became the first in a series of specifically targeted compounds directed against the cancer by design, and while these are usually expensive therapies, fewer side effects are incurred than with many other types of drugs precisely because they are targeted to the ways in which specific cancers evolve.

A host of targeted drug therapies has been developed since Gleevac was first identified, including Herceptin (or Traztuzimab, used for breast cancer), Cituximab (or Erbitux, used for head, neck, and colorectal cancers), and many others. These targeted therapies have ushered in a new era of "smart drug" developments that interfere with cancer-specific pathways identified in the laboratory as essential for the cell division and thriving of cancer.

To be sure, the history of cancer treatment is as old as the history of human cancers, but in the preceding centuries, better therapies with surgery, radiation, and, more recently, chemotherapies were produced. Very recently, new genetic insights have enabled us to understand why what has not worked did not do so, and why what works has worked, and to develop targeted therapies that focus on cancer cells and leave others alone. And as an evolutionary phenomenon, increasingly cancer is being treated as a chronic disease that may be not always be cured but increasingly may be manageable.

Development of Treatment Resistance

Two general types of resistance to anti-cancer treatments can be noted. One develops gradually over the course of treatment and it arises as a part of the evolution of the cancer in the body of the patient. In this case the development of resistance to the chemotherapy that is being administered is a result of newly acquired mutations of cancer cells. The second type of treatment resistance is the inherent property of (some) cancer types. Sometimes cancers are just resistant to the chemotherapy because therapeutic molecules cannot enter into the tumor. For example, pancreatic tumors are most often encapsulated by a "desmoplastic stroma" that limits the blood supply (which is carrying the chemotherapeutic molecules) to the tumor. This is a physical barrier that causes the cancer to be innately resistant to the drug.

There are many mechanisms for gradual induction of drug resistance, but the most common is a mutation that consists of an amplification of the gene known as MDR (multi-drug resistance). The MDR gene encodes the glycoprotein 100, a protein that functions as a transporter for different non-biological molecules (including drugs) from inside the cell to outside the cell. Gene amplification (which also occurs with some of the oncogenes, see elsewhere) is a process whereby a gene that is originally present in only a few copies in the cell becomes present in millions of copies all of which can code for the same protein. The process of gene amplification is one of the by-products of genomic instability in cancer (see chapter 3).

While any gene can be amplified though this process, selection pressure of chemotherapy provides the cells that have amplified MDR gene with an added survival (i.e. evolutionary) advantage. The net result is that the multiple copies of MDR gene make thousands of copies of the protein, which moves to the membrane of the cell and pumps out any chemotherapeutic drug that penetrated the cell membrane. This means that the chemotherapeutic agent, which is supposed to kill the tumor cell, leaks out of the cells that it was meant to kill through the use of the MDR gene encoding protein. This diverting of the chemotherapeutic drugs makes the tumor resistant to the drugs given to the patient to kill the tumor.

This distinctive type of enforced evolution of the tumor within the organism significantly impacts effectiveness of therapies. It makes the tumor able to ignore the chemotherapy. During the course of chemotherapy, the cells that amplify the MDR gene survive while the others are killed, again creating a unique natural selection scenario in the body for those cells that survive the best following chemotherapy administration. The tumor that evolves multi-drug resistance (through gene amplification or some other means) will be able to evade the anti-tumor therapy and thus avoid cell killing. Importantly, very often resistance to one drug applies to several other drug types as well.

While multi-drug resistance gene amplification is a common way in which cancer cells develop drug resistance, other mechanisms for drug and therapy resistance have also been identified. These mechanisms include the activation of endogenous scavengers for free radicals in tumor cells (free radicals damage DNA and lead to cell death) and activation of proteins that inactivate cellular pathways involved in metabolism of chemotherapeutic drugs that are critical for impact of the drug on cells. Drug resistance has been shown for a variety of different chemotherapeutic agents that target some growth factor receptor pathways, and drugs that modulate hormone therapies.

Radiation therapy is used to treat approximately 50 percent of all cancers, and resistance to radiation has also been documented in many tumors. Unlike resistance to drugs (which, as noted above, can mean as high as a thousandfold difference from the most sensitive to the most resistant cells), resistance to radiation is at most three- or fourfold between the most sensitive and the most resistant cells. The mechanisms of radiation resistance are more complex than the mechanisms of drug resistance and usually involve many genes instead of only one or two genes as occurs in drug resistance. In addition, there is rarely any cross-resistance between drugs and radiation, i.e., tumor cells that are drug resistant are not necessarily resistant to chemotherapy and vice-versa.

Resistance to radiation is often associated with changes in how quickly the cancer cells progress through the cell cycle and/or how efficiently DNA repair processes take place in cells following radiation exposure. Radiation resistance, although less dramatic than chemotherapy, can also limit the effectiveness of therapy. The distinctive evolution of radiation resistance during the course of radiotherapy and means of overcoming it are just now being exploited with therapeutic approaches.

Immune Therapies

Immune therapies are a collection of approaches that attempt to use either the innate immune system of the patient or immunologic substances from other organisms to fight cancer. There are three types of immune therapies that are generally used therapeutically. The goal of these therapies is to create an environment in the patient that is even more hostile for cancer evolution, that makes it even more difficult for the cancer to evolve in the patient. The first is a group of therapies known as cancer vaccines or cell-based therapies. In most cases, this approach consists of removing the immune cells from the patient with cancer and then mixing them with the tumor itself so that the cells develop an immune response to the tumor and can fight the tumor better. Most of these vaccines involve the activation of the patient's own immune cells so that they are better able to fight the cancer. While many experimental attempts were made for this type of vaccine, the only one that is currently in clinical use is Provenge (also called Spileucel-T), which is used for treatment of prostate cancer.[20]

The second type of immunologic anti-cancer therapy involves the use of "foreign," not made by the patient, antibodies. Antibodies are currently the most effective and commonly used form of immunotherapy, with clinically approved applications for a variety of different cancers. The antibody is a protein complex that is able to bind to specific target molecules, so-called antigens, and enable their attack by other components of the immune system leading to removal of antigens (together with larger structures they may be attached to) from the body. These antibodies are usually made against proteins uniquely present on the cell surface of the cancer cells but not on most normal cells. These antibodies can be coupled to a payload of chemotherapy or radiation and thus can deliver a "bomb" to the cancer cells.

The third type of immune therapy that is used in the United States, again engaging the patients' own immune system, is cytokine therapy. Cytokines are proteins produced by the body that regulate the immune system and thus can be used as agents to stimulate an anti-tumor immune response. The most commonly used classes of cytokines are interferons and interleukins. Interferons were originally discovered as substances that interfered with viral infections in the host, but have also been found to be effective in provoking an anti-tumor response. Interferons have been used successfully in treatment of some leukemias and also in melanomas. Interleukins are proteins that have a wide variety of different effects on the immune system. One of the most commonly used is Interleukin-2, which activates some white blood cells to develop anti-tumor activity, although the precise mechanism by which it works is not known. Interleukin-2 is used for treatment of some melanomas and also renal cell cancer.[21]

Much anti-cancer immunology research is ongoing with other immunostimulants that have come from a variety of different sources. BCG (bacillus Calmette-Guerin, a French name) was developed as a vaccine against tuberculosis that is prepared against the tuberculosis strain that causes the disease in the cows. Worldwide there is great variation on how this vaccine is used; in the United States it is rarely administered while in some countries of Europe it is given to all school children under the age of thirteen. Recently, BCG has become an effective treatment for some

20. Gardner et al., "Sipuleucel-T (Provenge)."
21. Dranoff, "Cytokines."

cancers, particularly bladder cancer. The vaccine is injected directly into the bladder and appears to stimulate a local immune response there. The exact mechanism of action in this case is not known, although some studies suggest that BCG is an immunostimulant that creates a strong environment that is hostile to cancer evolution. Overall, it has been successfully used to prevent bladder cancer recurrence in up to two-thirds of all bladder cancer patients.[22] It is also being exploited for a variety of other new experimental therapies that could lead to new promising approaches for treatment.

Complications in Cancer Treatment

An important consequence of most anti-cancer therapies is the possibility for the development of a second cancer unrelated to the first that is actually induced by the therapy itself. Most of the chemotherapeutic agents and the radiation that are used to treat cancer are also able to cause mutations that lead to cancer. While the incidences of this type of secondary cancers are often low, physicians reason that the risk of the secondary cancer is often a small price to pay for extending the life of the person who had cancer in the first place.

For radiation, the risk of secondary cancer is generally lower than it is for most chemotherapeutic agents, and for that reason radiation is used to treat well over half of cancers. In addition, secondary cancers from radiation usually occur somewhere near the treatment field, where the primary cancer was located and treated, and can therefore be prescreened more easily. For chemotherapeutic agents, the incidence of secondary cancers is somewhat higher and it can occur anywhere in the body, at distant sites. For example, in people treated for Hodgkin's disease (a tumor of the lymphoid system), the secondary cancer from chemotherapeutic drugs is often a leukemia, while for women treated for Hodgkin's with radiation, the secondary cancer is often breast cancer near the field where the person was irradiated.

There is also a different time course for induction of the cancer by chemotherapy vs. radiation. Leukemias from chemotherapy often occur within the first five years after treatment whereas, e.g., breast cancers from radiotherapy most often appear fifteen or more years later. These secondary cancers develop for two reasons: therapy itself creates an environment

22. One of the most important studies of the efficacy of BCG was reported by Lamm et al., "A Randomized Trial."

in the patient that is somewhat debilitated and permits a new cancer to evolve and at the same time therapy induces mutations that allow a new cancer to develop.

Summary

Cancer is not the incurable disease that it once was. In the past, there were few drugs that could be used to treat cancer, and most of these drugs had a single mechanism of action—to kill cells that were actively dividing. This approach for treatment is still successful and leads to good results for many different cancers. Recent years have seen the mushrooming of new therapies for fighting cancer, many of which have helped make cancer a disease people live with rather than a disease people die from.

These therapies include new approaches to radiation, a common modality that has been used successfully for almost a century to treat cancer, particularly when coupled with surgery and chemotherapy. New chemotherapeutic approaches have become available and continue to contribute new approaches for cancer treatment, giving hope for patients with those cancers that are difficult to treat. One concern with many of these therapies is that the tumor evolves in the patient over time, acquiring new mutations that make the cancer resistant to a therapy that was once successful lose its efficacy. Nevertheless, it has been through identifying evolutionary events in cancer itself that have enabled scientists and physicians to develop therapies that target the most important mutations in the disease.

To be sure, chance still drives the development of cancers, but we are increasingly able to "tame chance" through our development of treatment strategies that anticipate the evolutionary nature of their progression. "Chance favors the prepared mind," so, accordingly, scientific minds are preparing better and better ways to treat cancer.

Practical and Pastoral Bearings
of Chance, Necessity, and Love

Having summarized practical theological studies of all sorts as alike in offering theological interpretations for faithful understandings and wise practices of various situations faced by humanity,[23] we have put forward

23. See again Farley, "Interpreting Situations."

in this book a practical theology of the disease of cancer as a "situation" of all human being. Accordingly, we first described how cancer develops through the dynamics of evolution and then offered theological perspectives on its evolutionary unfolding. In aiming at the broad audience of all human beings, we noted that our inquiry distinguishes itself from the many helpful resources currently available focusing on pastoral care for persons with cancer and also for those who care about them.

However, in a previous study—"The Very Fiber of Our Being: A Pastoral Theology of Cancer and Evolution"—one of us, Leonard Hummel, explored the pastoral bearings of understanding cancer as a disease of evolution. During a year and a half of communal inquiry, Hummel and five congregational pastors explored, among other things, these questions:

> (1) How may God be preached, taught, and, in pastoral care, understood if the development of life and the development of cancers are linked by evolution? In addressing this one question, we considered these related ones: If God has created a world wherein the evolution of life makes possible the evolution of cancers, how may we understand and, thereby, witness to the goodness of God? (2) What does pastoral wisdom look like if cancers are something that, as evolutionary phenomena, sometimes can be changed and, at other times, cannot be? In addressing this particular question, we also considered the following ones: Are cancers as evolutionary phenomena something that we, in faith, are called on to accept? Are they something that we, in faith, may hope will not always be with us? What is pastoral practice that accepts this world with cancers in it and, also, hopes for something more?

The pastors in this study were four Lutheran ministers and one Episcopal priest serving congregations in Maryland, Pennsylvania, Minnesota, and Florida.[24] Prior to their initial gathering, they were provided with a general bibliography on cancer and religion, offered a half-day tutorial on basic cancer science, and, throughout the study, they reviewed three books dealing with the evolutionary nature of cancer. The pastors met with the project leader three times and completed two short papers and a summary report in order to address the questions above.

24. Pr. David Albertson, Living Grace Lutheran Church, Urbana, Maryland; Rev. Pam Fickenscher, Edina Community Lutheran Church, Edina, Minnesota; Rev. Stephen Herr, Christ Lutheran Church, Gettysburg, Pennsylvania; Rev. Kate Kelderman, Episcopal Church of Bethesda by the Sea, Palm Beach, Florida; Pr. Jean Kuebler, Big Spring United Lutheran Church, Newville, Pennsylvania.

What did this project reveal about a pastoral theology focused on the evolutionary nature of cancer's origins and outcomes? In her mid-project paper, one pastor, Jean Kuebler, observed that existential concerns about the chance and necessity of cancer arose among many in her congregation, herself included:

> In this particular congregational setting, we thought that . . . it would be more helpful and appropriate to focus on the existential implications of the fact that cancer is an evolutionary phenomenon. What if cancer is just some random thing that happens sometimes as part of the potential collateral damage of being human, and is not an act of God? What if the emergence of cancer (and its potential for resilient persistence and re-emergence) always contains an element of chance, and is not something that can be completely contained or controlled?

Upon review, it appears that all the pastors and many of their parishioners also sought ways to cope with and find consolation for existential issues brought on by this evolutionary disease. In one Lutheran congregation, the pastor reported how her congregation sought ways to build caring relationships and closeness amidst the existential "not-knowing" of how cancer would progress in any and all cases. In another Lutheran congregation, the pastor reported how he and his members sought to make meaning of cancer given its appearance as "something absurd." Pastor Kuebler reported that members of her congregation found some consolation for the above-noted existential dilemmas by meditating on the God of Job, but experienced more comfort through close and caring relationships with others. In an Episcopal parish in Florida, the pastor shared how members of her congregation achieved significant comfort by bringing extensive and well-researched theological meaning-making to cancer and also by learning more about the particulars of the disease process itself. And in a Pennsylvania congregation, the pastor shared how both some congregants found hope amidst, while others struggled with, the existential challenges of cancer's evolutionary nature.

These existential dimensions appeared in the pastors' reports that were focused on the two research questions. First, *how may God be preached, taught, and, in pastoral care, understood if the development of life and the development of cancers are linked by evolution?* Two pastors recounted that they conducted adult education sessions in which their congregants were able to situate evolutionary science about cancer within larger biblical and theological narratives of God's providential and redeeming love. In her summary report, one pastor claimed that many interpretative "wide lenses" may be brought to the phenomenon of cancer in order to make it theologically comprehensible. For example, having relied heavily on the theology of Teilhard de Chardin, this pastor found consolation in adopting the "wide-angle" perspective on cancer afforded by Teilhard's proposal that all things—including cancers—are being guided toward the "Omega" point of the Cosmic Christ. And both of these pastors reported that they and their parishioners experienced the actively caring cancer support groups in their congregations as signs of God's love and faithfulness here and now and amidst the turmoil of cancer's evolutionary development.

And while she noted limits to the consoling effects of educational inquiry, Kuebler recounted how biblical text study focusing on human suffering aided their reflections on cancer's evolutionary nature. "Their consensus was that cancer is something that just happens, that it is a side effect of being human, and that cancer is not particularly God's idea or God's will. They 'got it' that God could be present in the silent accompaniment of Job's friends, in the faithful persistence of Job's wife, and in the visits and gifts of Job's friends and neighbors at the end of his trials."

As part of his more broadly focused ministry of outreach through YouTube presentations, one pastor publicly reflected on the science of cancer and the existential predicaments posed by its evolutionary development. On the other hand, having researched the chance and necessity of cancer, this same pastor concluded that "Understanding biology and evolution have greatly improved my understanding of cancer and also of the professional and medical experiences of many more people in the congregation. Cancer is no longer a mysterious devil." Another pastor reported that comprehending cancer as an evolutionary phenomenon helped him to grasp more particulars of its processes. However, he also noted that a few congregants did struggle to reconcile the evolutionary principles contained in this understanding with faith in a providential God.

Secondly, *what does pastoral wisdom look like if cancers are something that, as evolutionary phenomena, sometimes can be changed, and at other times, cannot be?*

All the participating pastors reported that pastoral wisdom included an appreciation for the enterprise of basic cancer science—for not only its locating the place of cancer within all life but also its contribution to more effective cancer treatments in many lives. Similarly, they claimed that comprehending aspects of cancer science would make them wiser in caring for those with the disease, e.g., "just as understanding the medicine around cardiac care helps one minister better to hear patients, understanding cancers, the research that is being done, helps one minister to parishioners." And Kuebler's suggestion that scientific findings be employed to help prevent occurrences of cancer was affirmed by all other pastors: "I guess pastoral wisdom also needs to speak law—encourage individuals to stop smoking. Encourage individuals as they make choices for an active lifestyle and a healthy diet."

While there was consensus about the need to better understand the nature of cancer and also to care for those with the disease, there was not complete agreement about how to reconcile faith in God and cancer's evolutionary nature. One pastor began her final report with this clear claim: "In the many conversations shared through this past year the goodness of God was never questioned. Regardless of the evolutionary nature of cancer and the pain it causes, God is good." However, another noted a disjunction between theological insights one might endorse and existential angst one might experience:

> The chaos and chance built into the nature of life on earth is bearable when told from the God's eye view of Job 38, or even from the microscopic view of the wonder of strangely mutated DNA. . . . But being part of the natural chaos of life while healthy is very different from being victim of the natural chaos of life. People do not easily find a way to come to terms with God and the world when their world has fallen apart.

How, then, do these findings of congregational pastoral care relate to other conclusions about pastoral care for cancer? They confirm the centrality of "the existential issues that challenge people with cancer" as Jann Alredge-Clanton details them in her now classic work, *Counseling People with Cancer*. "The uncertainty surrounding this disease is one of the most formidable challenges. Living with the unknown creates more anxiety for some people than any diagnosis or prognosis concerning their cancer. . . . All the waiting with this disease creates stress and challenges hope."[25]

And how do they compare with our own exploration of cancer and evolution? They echo the existential concerns presaged by Monod and articulated by Greaves concerning the linkage of life with the enduring realities reality of cancer. At the same time, most experiences of these pastors

25. Aldredge-Clanton, *Counseling People with Cancer*, 7.

and their people also appear to be in communion with Peacocke's affirmation of faith in his final days. To be sure, Peacocke faced squarely the existential challenges brought to human being—his own, included—by the dynamisms of chance and necessity. At the same time, he was able to proffer an account of divine presence amidst these evolutionary forces as they expressed themselves in the disease of cancer.

Similarly, in the congregation where some wrestled with cancer and evolution, the response of their pastor epitomized the pastoral response of all of them: "If cancer is evolutionary and based on chance, it does provide the opportunity to speak a Word of God's incarnated presence and love in the midst of a creation where chance and randomness are present." That is to say, the pastors understood themselves called to minister to all amidst the questions and concerns generated by the chance and necessity of cancer.

As noted, all of the pastors concerned themselves with making meaning of and coping with the evolutionary features of the disease of cancer. That is, in their consideration of pastoral activities and pastoral wisdom, each pastor sought out theological resources to interpret cancer's evolutionary development. Given the pervasively empathic concern by the church for those with cancer, this project demonstrated evolutionary theory need not be too hot or too cold for a suffering world and a church that cares about their suffering.

Final Remarks

As we stated in the introduction, our intent throughout this book also has been to demonstrate that theological reflection on evolutionary theory may assist us in developing faithful understandings and wise responses to the phenomenon of cancer. Accordingly, we have meditated on the goodness of God even as creation and cancer are bound together. We also have described how we may hope for more—both now and always—given that the ways cancers occur and unfold sometimes may be changed. And we have claimed that the love of God may be discerned in these ways:

> Through their research, scientific "communities of inquiry" strive to understand and, increasingly succeed at understanding the evolutionary nature of cancers. The efforts of these communities, carried out by persons both of faith and of no faith, may evidence the love of God at work in, with and under the evolution of cancers.

Since cancer is the inevitable consequence of human evolution, at some level it is a consequence of being evolving human beings and is of necessity required for our existence. Based on this, it is clear that cancer is a consequence that humanity must face in order to be evolving creatures that can survive in this world; as such, then, each person that suffers from cancer is paying the price for humanity's evolution and therefore deserves our love and support. Our responsibility as human persons is that we must care for those with cancer because they are suffering the consequences in place for all humanity; their disease is the disease of all humanity, and their suffering is the suffering of all humanity. We have a responsibility of love, care, and ease of pain and suffering that is a needed consequence of our responsibility to others who are suffering on behalf of all of humanity.

We also have proposed the love of God is present in this way:

> Through symbols and stories about the chance and necessity of the disease of cancer, we have the ability to construct meanings about that evolutionary phenomenon. God may work in, with and under these constructions to reveal and make real God's love for this world with cancers in it.

Accordingly, we conclude by calling on theologians, lay and professional, to find even more ways to discern the presence of love—divine and human—amidst the evolutionary development of cancers. Given that the very act of religious reflection on the chance and necessity of cancers is one of the ways in which such love may be at work in the world, it behooves persons of faith to craft even more theologies regarding the evolution of cancers.

Bibliography

Alberts, Bruce, et al. *Molecular Biology of the Cell.* 6th ed. New York: Garland Science, 2014.

Aldredge-Clanton, Jann. *Counseling People with Cancer. Counseling and Pastoral Theology.* Louisville: Westminster John Knox, 1998.

Ayala, Francis J. "Chance and Necessity: Adaptation and Novelty in Evolution." In *An Evolving Dialogue: Theological and Scientific Perspectives on Evolution,* edited by James B. Miller, 231–62. Harrisburg, PA: Trinity, 2001.

American Cancer Society. www.cancer.org.

Baum, Christopher, et al. "Chance or Necessity? Insertional Mutagenesis in Gene Therapy and Its Consequences." *Molecular Therapy* 9:1 (January 2004) 5–13.

Bede. *Ecclesiastical History of the English People.* London: Penguin, 1990.

Benzein, Eva, et al. "The Meaning of the Lived Experience of Hope in Patients with Cancer in Palliative Home Care." *Palliative Medicine* 15:2 (March 2001) 117–26.

Berger, Michael F., et al. "Melanoma Genome Sequencing Reveals Frequent PREX2 Mutations." *Nature* 485:7399 (May 2012) 502–6.

Blagden, Sarah P., and Anne E. Willis. "The Biological and Therapeutic Relevance of mRNA Translation in Cancer." *Nature Reviews Clinical Oncology* 8 (May 2011) 280–91.

Bonhoeffer, Dietrich. *Letters and Papers from Prison.* Edited by Eberhard Bethge. Translated by R. H. Fuller. New York: Macmillan, 1972.

Bonnet, Dominique, and John E. Dick. "Human Acute Myeloid Leukemia is Organized as a Hierarchy that Originates from a Primitive Hematopoietic Cell." *Nature Medicine* 3:7 (1997) 730–37.

Bonting, Sjoerd. *Chaos Theology: A Revised Creation Theology.* Toronto: Novalis, 2002.

Boyle, Peter, and Bernard Levin, eds. *The World Cancer Report 2008.* Lyon: International Agency for Cancer Research, 2008.

Brown, Nelson E., and Philip W. Hinds. "Tumor Suppressor Genes." In *The Molecular Basis of Cancer* 4th ed., edited by John Mendelsohn et al., 35–46. Philadelphia: Elsevier, 2015.

Callaway, Ewen. "NIH Director Explains HeLa Agreement." *Nature News* (August 7, 2013). http://www.nature.com/news/nih-director-explains-hela-agreement-1.13521.

Campbell, Bernard. *Human Evolution.* 4th ed. New York: Aldine, 1998.

Campbell-Reed, Eileen R. "Baptist Clergywomen's Narratives: Reinterpreting the Southern Baptist Convention Schism." In *Pastoral Bearings: Lived Religion and Pastoral Theology,* edited by Jane F. Maynard et al., 143–78. Lanham, MD: Lexington, 2010.

Capasso, Luigi L. "Antiquity of Cancer." *International Journal of Cancer* 113 (2005) 2–13.

Carrol, Sean B. *Brave Genius: A Scientist, a Philosopher, and Their Daring Adventures from the French Resistance to the Nobel Prize.* New York: Crown, 2013.

Carter, R. L. "Infectious Mononucleosis: Model for Self-Limiting Lymphoproliferation." *The Lancet* 305:7911 (1975) 846–49.

Chang, David K., et al. "Mining the Genomes of Exceptional Responders." *Nature Reviews Cancer* 14:5 (2014) 291–92.

Children's Oncology Group. www.childrensoncologygroup.org.

Chung, Johnathan C., et al. "Four-dimensional Transcatheter Intra-arterial Perfusion MR Imaging Before and After Uterine Artery Embolization in the Rabbit VX2 Tumor Model." *Journal of Magnetic Resonance Imaging* 31 (2010) 1137–43.

Clayton, Philip. Introduction to *All That Is: A Naturalistic Faith for the Twenty-First Century,* by Arthur Peacocke. Edited by Philip Clayton. Minneapolis: Fortress, 2007.

Clevers, Hans. "The Cancer Stem Cell: Premises, Promises and Challenges." *Nature Medicine* 17:3 (March 2011) 313–19.

Clow, Barbara. *Negotiating Disease: Power and Cancer Care, 1900–1950.* Toronto: McGill-Queens University Press, 2001.

Cocco, P., et al. "Lung Cancer among Silica-Exposed Workers: The Quest for Truth between Chance and Necessity." *La Medicina del lavoro* 98:1 (2007) 3–17.

Couture Pamela. *Blessed Are the Poor? Women's Poverty, Family Policy, and Practical Theology.* Nashville: Abindgon, 1991.

Crenshaw, James L. *Old Testament Wisdom: An Introduction.* Louisville: Westminster John Knox, 2010.

Darwin, Charles. *The Descent of Man, and Selection in Relation to Sex.* New York: Hurst & Co., 1996.

————. *On the Origin of Species.* Oxford: Oxford University Press, 2009.

Dehart, Paul J. *Beyond the Necessary: Trinitarian Faith and Philosophy in the Thought of Eberhard Jüngel.* Atlanta: Scholars, 1999.

De Duve, Christian. "Thoughts of a Senior Scientist: Chance and Necessity Revisited." *Cellular and Molecular Life Sciences* 64 (2007) 3149–58.

De Morgan, Sophia Elizabeth, ed. *A Budget of Paradoxes.* London: Longmans, Green, and Co., 1872.

Dranoff, Glenn. "Cytokines in Cancer Pathogenesis and Cancer Therapy." *Nature Reviews Cancer* 4:1 (Jan 2004) 11–22.

Eldridge, Michael. "*Anhedonia* and the Broken World: William James and Gabriel Marcel on Vagueness and Mystery." Department of Philosophy, University of North Carolina, Charlotte. http://www.philosophy.uncc.edu/mleldrid/SAAP/USC/TP33.html.

"'The Emperor of All Maladies' and Louis Menand." http://themargin1.wordpress.com/2011/06/20/the-emperor-of-all-maladies-and-louis-menand/.

Evangelical Lutheran Church in America. "A Social Statement on Genetics, Faith, and Responsibility." http://www.elca.org/Faith/Faith-and-Society/Social-Statements/Genetics?_ga=1.205455440.1946099690.1422410977.

Farley, Edward. *Divine Empathy: A Theology of God*. Minneapolis: Fortress, 1996.

———. *Good and Evil: Interpreting a Human Condition*. Minneapolis: Fortress, 1990.

———. "Interpreting Situations: An Inquiry into the Nature of Practical Theology." In *The Blackwell Reader in Practical and Pastoral Theology*, edited by James Woodward and Stephen Pattison, 118–27. Hoboken, NJ: Wiley/Blackwell, 2000.

———. "Some Preliminary Thoughts on a Practical Theology of Cancer." Photocopy, Vanderbilt Divinity School, Vanderbilt University.

"Fiber." In *American Heritage Dictionary of the English Language*. 5th ed. Accessed June 13, 2016. http://www.thefreedictionary.com/fiber.

Fitzgerald, Patrick J. *From Demons and Evil Spirits to Cancer Genes: The Development of Concepts Concerning the Causes of Cancer and Carcinogenesis*. Washington, DC: American Registry of Pathology, 2000.

Flint, Jane S., et al. *Principles of Virology*. 2 vols. 3rd ed. Washington, DC: ASM, 2000.

Franco, Eduardo L., et al. "Epidemiologic Evidence and Human Papillomavirus Infection as a Necessary Cause of Cervical Cancer." *Journal of the National Cancer Institute* 91:6 (March 1999), 506–11.

Futreal, P. Andrew, et al. "A Census of Human Cancer Genes." *Nature Reviews Cancer* 4 (2004) 177–83.

Futuyma, Douglas J. *Evolutionary Biology*. Sunderland, MA: Sinauer Associates, 1997.

Gardner, Thomas, et al. "Sipuleucel-T (Provenge) Autologous Vaccine Approved for Treatment of Men with Asymptomatic or Minimally Symptomatic Castrate-Resistant Metastatic Prostate Cancer." *Human Vaccines & Immunotherapeutics* 8:4 (April 2012) 534–39.

Greaves, Mel. *Cancer: The Evolutionary Legacy*. Oxford: Oxford University Press, 2000.

GenBank. www.ncbi.nim/nih.gov/genbank.

Hacking, Ian. *The Taming of Chance*. Cambridge: Cambridge University Press, 1990.

Hanahan, Douglas, and Robert Weinberg. "The Hallmarks of Cancer." *Cell* 100 (2000) 57–70.

———. "Hallmarks of Cancer: The Next Generation." *Cell* 144 (2011) 646–74.

Hegel, Georg Wilhelm Friedrich. *Lectures on the Philosophy of Religion vol. III: The Consummate Religion*. Edited by Peter C. Hodgson. Translated by R. F. Brown, et al. New York: Oxford University Press, 1985.

Hoption Cann, S. A., et al. "Spontaneous Regression: A Hidden Treasure Buried in Time." *Medical Hypotheses* 58 (February 2002) 115–19.

Howe, Susan. *Pierce-Arrow*. New York: New Directions, 1999.

Huang, Sui. "Cancer as Developmental Disease: Chance and Necessity in Networks Dynamics During Somatic Evolution of Cancer Cells." Lecture, University of Cambridge, Cambridge, UK, February 1, 2011.

———. "On the Intrinsic Inevitability of Cancer: From Foetal to Fatal Attraction." *Seminars in Cancer Biology* 21:3 (June 2011) 183–99.

Hummel, Leonard M. *Clothed in Nothingness: Consolation for Suffering*. Minneapolis: Fortress, 2003.

———. "A Thing That Cannot and Can Be Changed: Teaching a Practical Theology of Cancer." Report for the Wabash Center for Teaching and Learning in Theology and Religion, Crawfordsville, IN, 2003.

Jackson, Kathyjo A., et al. "Regeneration of Ischemic Cardiac Muscle and Vascular Endothelium by Adult Stem Cells." *Journal of Clinical Investigation* 107:11 (2001) 1395–1402.

Jackson, Robert. "Saint Peregrine, O.S.M.—The Patron Saint of Cancer Patients." *Canadian Medical Association Journal* 111 (October 19, 1974) 824.

Jacob, François, and Jacques Monod. "Genetic Regulatory Mechanisms in the Synthesis of Proteins." *Journal of Molecular Biology* 3 (1961) 318–56.

"Jacques Monod—Facts." http://www.nobelprize.org/nobel_prizes/medicine/laureates/1965/monod.html.

James, William. *The Principles of Psychology*. Cambridge, MA: Harvard University Press, 1981.

————. *The Will to Believe and Other Essays in Popular Philosophy*. New York: Dover, 1956.

Jarus, Owen. "Egyptian Mummy Had Cancer, Diabetes, Study Suggests." *The Huffington Post*, April 27, 2012. http://www.huffingtonpost.com/2012/04/27/ancient-egyptian-mummy-hand-schuller-christian-disease_n_1459929.html.

Judson, Horace Freeland. *The Eighth Day of Creation: Makers of the Revolution in Biology*. New York: Simon and Schuster, 1979.

Jüngel, Eberhard. *God as the Mystery of the World: On the Foundation of the Theology of the Crucified One in the Dispute between Theism and Atheism*. Translated by Darrel L. Gruder. Grand Rapids: Eerdmans, 1983.

Keightley, Peter D. "Rates and Fitness Consequences of New Mutations in Humans." *Genetics* 190:2 (February 2012) 295–304.

King, Mary-Claire, et al. "Breast and Ovarian Cancer Risks Due to Inherited Mutations in BRCA1 and BRCA2." *Science* 302:5645 (October 2003) 643–46.

Kitano, Hiroaki. "Cancer as a Robust System: Implications for Anticancer Therapy." *Nature Reviews Cancer* 4 (March 2004) 227–35.

Knudson, Alfred G. "Mutation and Cancer: Statistical Study of Retinoblastoma." *Proceedings of the National Academy of the Sciences of the United States of America* 68:4 (1971) 820–23.

Lamm, Donald L., et al. "A Randomized Trial of Intravesical Doxorubicin and Immunotherapy with Bacille Calmette-Guerin for Transitional-Cell Carcinoma of the Bladder." *The New England Journal of Medicine* 325:2 (1991) 1205–9.

Landry, Jonathan, et al. "The Genomic and Transcriptomic Landscape of a HeLa Cell Line." *G3* (Bethesda) 3:8 (August 2013) 1213–24.

Lehnert, Shirley, ed. *Biomolecular Action of Ionizing Radiation*. Medical Physics and Biomedical Engineering. New York: Taylor & Francis, 2007.

Lewandowski, Robert J., et al. "Functional Magnetic Resonance Imaging in an Animal Model of Pancreatic Cancer." *World Journal of Gastroenterology* 16:26 (2010) 3292–98.

Lodish, Harvey, et al. *Molecular Cell Biology*. 6th ed. New York: W. H. Freeman, 2007.

Luther, Martin. *Luther's Works vol 14: Selected Psalms III*. Edited by Jaroslav Pelikan. St. Louis: Concordia, 1958.

Manchester Keith L. "Theodor Boveri and the Origin of Malignant Tumors." *Trends in Cell Biology* 5:10 (October 1995) 384–87.

Marcel, Gabriel. *Homo Viator: Introduction to a Metaphysic of Hope*. Translated by Emma Craufurd. New York: Harper and Row, 1962.

————. *The Philosophy of Existentialism*. Translated by Manya Harari. New York: Carol, 1995.

Martin, Ralph P. *A Hymn of Christ: Philippians 2:5–11 in Recent Interpretation & in the Setting of Early Christian Worship*. Downers Grove, IL: InterVarsity, 1997.

Merlo, Lauren M. F., et al. "Cancer as an Evolutionary and Ecological Process." *Nature Reviews Cancer* 6 (December 2006) 924–35.

Moltmann, Jürgen. *Science and Wisdom*. Translated by Margaret Kohl. Minneapolis: Fortress, 2003.

Monod, Jacques. *Chance and Necessity: An Essay on the Natural Philosophy of Modern Biology*. Translated by Austryn Wainhouse. New York: Alfred A. Knopf, 1971.

————. *Lecon inaugurale: faite le Vendredi 3 novembre 1967*. Nogent-le-Rotrou: Daupeley-Govenereur.

Moss, Lenny. "From Representational Preformationism to the Epigenesis of Openness to the World? Reflections on a New Vision of the Organism." *Annals of the New York Academy of Sciences* 981 (2002) 219–29.

Mukherjee, Siddhartha. *The Emperor of All Maladies: A Biography of Cancer*. New York: Scribner, 2010.

Murchison, Elizabeth P., et al. "Transmissible Dog Cancer Genome Reveals the Origin and History of an Ancient Cell Lineage." *Science* 343:6169 (January 2014) 437–40.

Murphy, George L. *The Cosmos in the Light of the Cross*. Rev. ed. Harrisburg, PA: Trinity, 2003.

Naugler, Christopher T. "Population Genetics of Cancer Cell Clones: Possible Implications of Cancer Stem Cells." *Theoretical Biology and Medical Modelling* 7:1 (October, 2010) 42.

"NIH, Lacks Family Reach Understanding to Share Genomic Data of HeLa Cells." August 7, 2013. https://www.nih.gov/news-events/news-releases/nih-lacks-family-reach-understanding-share-genomic-data-hela-cells.

O'Connell, J. F., et al. "Grandmothering and the Evolution of Homo erectus." *Journal of Human Evolution* 36:5 (May 1999) 461–85.

Olson, James S. *Bathsheba's Breast: Women, Cancer, and History* (Baltimore: Johns Hopkins Press, 2002).

Orlic, Donald, et al. "Bone Marrow Cells Regenerate Infarcted Myocardium." *Nature* 410 (2001) 701–5.

Pack, George T. "St. Peregrine, O.S.M.—The Patron Saint of Cancer Patients." *CA: A Cancer Journal for Clinicians* 17 (1967) 183–4.

Page, Ruth. *God and the Web of Creation*. London: SCM, 1996.

Patterson, James T. *The Dread Disease: Cancer and Modern American Culture*. Cambridge, MA: Harvard University Press, 1987.

Peacocke, Arthur R. *All That Is: A Naturalistic Faith for the Twenty-First Century*. Edited by Philip Clayton. Minneapolis: Fortress, 2007.

————. "Chance and Law." In *Chaos and Complexity: Scientific Perspectives on Divine Action*, edited by Robert John Russell et al., 123–46. Rome: The Vatican Observatory Foundation, 1995.

————. "Chance and the Life Game." *Zygon* 14:4 (December 1979) 301–22.

————. "Chance and Necessity in the Life-Game." *Trends in Biochemical Sciences* 2:5 (1977) N99-N100.

————. "Chance, Potentiality and God." *The Modern Churchman* 17:1 (New Series 1973) 13–23.

————. *Evolution: The Disguised Friend of Faith?* Philadelphia: Templeton Foundation, 2004.

————. "God's Action in the Real World." *Zygon* 26:4 (December 1991) 455–76.

————. *Theology for a Scientific Age: Being and Becoming—Natural, Divine, and Human.* Rev. ed. Minneapolis: Fortress, 1993.

————. "Welcoming the 'Disguised Friend'—Darwinism and Divinity." In *Intelligent Design and Its Critics: Philosophical, Theological, and Scientific Perspectives*, edited by Robert T. Pennock, 471–86. Cambridge, MA: MIT Press, 2001.

Peirce, Charles Sanders. *Collected Papers of Charles Sanders Peirce.* Edited by Charles Hartshorne and Paul Weiss. Cambridge, MA: Harvard University Press, 1932–1958.

Peters, Karl E. *Dancing with the Sacred: Evolution, Ecology, and God.* Harrisburg, PA: Trinity, 2002.

Peters, Ted, and Martinez Hewlett. *Evolution from Creation to New Creation: Conflict, Conversation, and Convergence.* Nashville: Abindgon, 2003.

Polkinghorne, John. "Does God Interact with His Suffering World?" James Gregory Lecture. University of St. Andrews. October 9, 2008.

————. "Science and Theology in the Twenty-First Century." *Zygon* 35:4 (2000) 941–53.

"Prayer to St. Peregrine." http://www.ewtn.com/Devotionals/novena/peregrine.htm.

Rather, J. R. *The Genesis of Cancer: A Study in the History of Ideas.* Baltimore: Johns Hopkins University Press, 1978.

"Researchers Find Cancer in Ancient Egyptian Mummy." *USA Today*, January 29, 2012. http://usatoday30.usatoday.com/tech/science/discoveries/story/2012-01-29/egypt-mummy-cancer/52869884/1.

Risch, Neil. "The Genetic Epidemiology of Cancer: Interpreting Family and Twin Studies and Their Implications for Molecular Genetic Approaches." *Cancer Epidemiology, Biomarkers and Prevention* 10 (July 2001) 733–41.

Rolston III, Holmes. "Naturalizing and Systematizing Evil." In *Is Nature Ever Evil? Religion, Science and Value*, edited by Willem B. Drees, 67–86. London: Routledge, 2003.

Russell, Robert John. "The Groaning of Creation: Does God Suffer with All Life?" In *The Evolution of Evil*, edited by Gaymon Bennet et al., 120–42. Religion, Theologie und Naturwissenschaft/Religion, Theology, and Natural Science. Göttingen: Vandenhoeck & Ruprecht, 2008.

Schaller, Janet E. "Resisting Stares and Stereotypes—Affirming Life." In *Pastoral Bearings: Lived Religion and Pastoral Theology*, edited by Jane F. Maynard et al., 121–42. Lanham, MD: Lexington, 2010.

Science & Technology Review (May 1997). https://www.llnl.gov/str/pdfs/05_97.pdf.

Skloot, Rebecca. *The Immortal Life of Henrietta Lacks.* London: Macmillan, 2010.

Smith, John E. *The Spirit of American Philosophy.* Albany, NY: SUNY Press, 1983.

Smith, John Maynard, and Eörs Szathmáry. *The Origins of Life: From the Birth of Life to the Origin of Language.* Oxford: Oxford University Press, 2000.

Smithers, D. W. "Cancer an Attack on Cytologism." *Lancet* 279:7228 (March 1962) 493–99.

Southgate, Christopher. "Creation as 'Very Good' and 'Groaning in Travail': An Exploration in Evolutionary Theodicy." In *The Evolution of Evil*, edited by Gaymon Bennet et al., 53–86. Religion, Theologie und Naturwissenschaft/Religion, Theology, and Natural Science. Göttingen: Vandenhoeck & Ruprecht, 2008.

Spindler, Stephen R. "Rapid and Reversible Induction of the Longevity, Anticancer and Genomic Effects of Caloric Restriction." *Mechanisms of Ageing and Development* 126:9 (September 2005) 960–66.

Stanier, R. Y. "Obituary: Jacques Monod, 1910–1976." *Journal of General Microbiology* 101 (1977) 1–12.

Steiner, George. "Chance and Necessity." *New York Times Book Review* (November 21, 1971) 5.

Thomas, Rachel, et al. "Extensive Conservation of Genomic Imbalance in Canine Transmissible Venereal Tumors (CTVT) Detected by Microarray-Based CGH Analysis." *Chromosome Research* 17:7 (2009) 927–34.

Thompson, Deanna. *Hoping for More, Having Cancer, Talking Faith, and Accepting Grace.* Eugene, OR: Cascade, 2012.

Torrance, Thomas F. *Divine and Contingent Order.* Oxford: Oxford University Press, 1981.

———. *Reality and Scientific Theology.* Edinburgh: Scottish Academic, 1985.

Van Speybroeck, Linda. "From Epigenesis to Epigenetics: The Case of C. H. Waddington." *Annals of the New York Academy of Sciences* 981 (2002) 61–81.

Von Rad, Gerhard. *Wisdom in Israel.* Translated by James D. Martin. Nashville: Abingdon, 1972.

Waddington, Conrad Hal. "The Epigenotype." *Endeavour* 1 (1942) 18–20.

Waggoner, Ben. "Robert Hooke." http://www.ucmp.berkeley.edu/history/hooke.html.

Wahl, Linda M., and David C. Krakauer. "Models of Experimental Evolution: The Role of Genetic Chance and Selective Necessity." *Genetics* 156 (November 2000) 1437–48.

Wangerin, Walter, Jr. *Letters from the Land of Cancer.* Grand Rapids: Zondervan, 2010.

Weiss, Leonard. "Early Concepts of Cancer." *Cancer Metastasis Reviews* 19 (2000) 205–17.

Wikipedia, s. v. "Genetic Drift." Last modified June 20, 2016. https://en.wikipedia.org/wiki/Genetic_drift.

———, s. v. "Lepus Cornutus." Last Modified June 26, 2016. https://en.wikipedia.org/wiki/Lepus_cornutus.

Wildman, Wesley. "Incongruous Goodness, Perilous Beauty, Disconcerting Truth: Ultimate Reality and Suffering In Nature." In *Physics and Cosmology: Scientific Perspectives on the Problem of Natural Evil*, edited by Robert J. Russell et al., 267–96. Vatican City: Vatican Observatory, 2008.

Williams, George C. "Pleitropy, Natural Selection, and the Evolution of Senescence." *Evolution* 11:4 (1957) 398–411.

Wilson, David Sloan. *Darwin's Cathedral: Evolution, Religion, and the Nature of Society.* Chicago: University of Chicago Press, 2002.

Woglum, William H. "Cancer, the Scourge of God." *The Atlantic Monthly* 141 (June 1928) 806–12.

Woloschak, Gayle. *Beauty and Unity in Creation: The Evolution of Life.* Minneapolis: Light & Life, 1996.

———. "Chance and Necessity in Arthur Peacocke's Scientific Work." *Zygon* 43:1 (March 2008) 75–87.

Yarbro Collins, Adela. "Psalms, Philippians 2:6–11, and the Origins of Christology." *Biblical Interpretation* 11:3 (2003) 361–72.

Author Index

Note: page numbers with "n" refer to notes; those with "f" refer to figures.

Subject Index

acceptance. *See also* faithful understandings; evolutionary theology of cancer
  as *Gelassenheit* (letting-be), 91–93
  as response to cancer, 6–7, 117–19, 92, 122, 141, 150
  of suffering, and recognition of God's will, 79, 120
  and accepting cancer as one of God's creations, 81–82, 91
adult stem cells, 30–32
agape (love). *See* love, God's
American Cancer Society, 18n11
amyotrophic lateral sclerosis (ALS, Lou Gehrig's disease), 66
ancient world, understandings of cancer in, 3–4, 60
Animal Qvarvpedia et Reptilia (Terra) (Hoefnagel), 25
animals
  cancers in, 19, 25, 56, 63
  research using, 18, 24, 32–33, 63–64, 69
antibody therapies, 162
apoptosis (programmed cell death), 27, 112, 160
asymptote figure, as metaphor for effects of God's love, 131, 131f
ataxia-telangietasia (AT), 67

atheistic perspectives
  and Jüngel's understanding of God's hidden purposefulness, 143
  and Monod's views of chance and necessity, 140
  and scientific inquiry, 137–38
Ayurvedic writings, India, 4

bacillus Calmette-Guerin (BCG) treatment, 162–63
Bede, Adam, 152–53
beliefs, impact on reality, 114–15
benign tumors, 28, 51
"The Biological and Therapeutic Relevance of mRNA Translation in Cancer" (Blagden and Willis), 123
biological evolution. *See also* evolutionary theology of cancer; genes, genomes
  characteristics, 54–56
  and freedom from disease in an evolved world, 102–3
  mutation and DNA repair, 57, 66
  Peirce's analysis, 129–132, 131f
  population level impacts, 59–60
  role of chance and necessity, 56–57
Bishop, J. Michael, 83, 139
bladder cancer treatment, 162–63

DNA *(continued)*
 Peacocke's discoveries related to, 124
 replication, as error-prone process,
  20–21, 58–59
dominant oncogenes, 40–41, 44

Earle, Henry, 36
empathy, God's, trusting in, 82
The Emperor of All Maladies: A Biography of Cancer (Mukherjee), 4–5, 116
energy metabolism by cancer cells, 27–28
environmental exposures
 cancers associated with, 25–26, 35
 limiting/controlling risks from, 113
epigenesis
 defined, 101n8
 Peters's construct, 101
epigenetic changes
 defined, 46
 and gene methylation, 46–47
 and histones, 47
 microRNAs, 47–48
Epstein-Barr virus, 23–24
"An Essay in Interpretation" (Peacocke), 150
Evangelical Lutheran Church, Social Statement on Genetics, 112
Evolutionary Biology (Futuyma), 54n1
evolutionary theology of cancer. *See also* creation/recreation, God's; kenosis; love, God's
 as evidence of divine love, 145–46
 basic precepts, 135–36
 and biological evolution, 7, 54–55, 59–60, 118–19, 135–36
 and cancer as manifestation of God's hidden work, 127, 142–45
 and the complexity of cancer, 138
 and acceptance of all God's creations, 81, 93n40, 96–99
 and faithful understandings of disease, x, 5–7, 85, 88–91, 93–95, 109–10, 137–38, 153, 156–58, 165–69

and genetic change/mutation as essential to existence, 10, 81, 117–18, 139, 152, 160
 Hummel's perspective, 135
 and the interplay of chance and necessity, 121–22, 126–27, 165
 Monod's perspective, 133–34
 Peacocke's perspective, 134–35
 Peirce's perspective, 135
 and reconciling acceptance and hope, 100, 118–19
 and understandings of God's love, 140–42
 understanding through communities of inquiry, 7, 156–58
 value of, for caregivers, 8
 understanding through scientific inquiry, 137–38
exposures, modulators of, 2f

faithful understandings. *See also* evolutionary theology of cancer; hope
 defined, x, 5
 sustaining, in light of experience of cancer, 78, 85, 88–89, 93–95
Farley, Edward
 and acceptance of all of creation, 96–97
 acceptance of paradox, randomness and disorder, 81
 definition of practical theology, 3
 and faithful understanding of cancer, 85, 88–89
 "magic land" envisioned by, 100–101
 on suffering as intrinsic to existence, 80–81, 104
Feuerbach, Ludwig, 143
"fiber of being" metaphor
 applicability to cancer cells, 13–15, 77
 defined, 14
 and responses to cancer, 117
food additives, cancers associated with, 25
Futuyma, Douglas J., 54n1, 55

gamma rays, cancers associated with, 26
Gelassenheit (letting-be), 91–93
GenBank, 65, 65n11

Necessity in Arthur Be